PREVENTING CANCER

HELPING TO CURE CANCER

CRITICAL LIFE-SAVING CANCER THERAPIES – NOT PRESCRIBED WITH CONVENTIONAL CANCER TREATMENT

DR. MERLE LOUDON

Preventing Cancer: Helping to Cure Cancer
First edition, published 2021

By Dr. Merle Loudon
Cover design by Reprospace.com

Copyright © 2021, Dr. Merle Loudon

Paperback Edition ISBN-13: 978-1-952685-07-1

All information in this book is for informational purposes only. It should not be interpreted as medical or health treatment.

If any supplement, nutrient, food, remedy, or dosage of supplements are mentioned or
written, do not rely on any of this information as medical treatment or medical advice.
Any dosages may vary and should be affirmed with your physician or naturopath. Before using any advice, treatment, dosages, or medical content, you should consult with
a licensed medical physician or health provider. This book's information is believed to
be accurate and sound, based on the best and latest information available. That does
not mean that the reader should not consult with a licensed health professional.

Before or when using any information, taking any supplements, remedies, or food
mentioned in this book, always check and get your physician's advice or naturopath. If
you have any questions or concerns before starting or modifying any cancer treatment,
do not rely on this information without your physician's advice or treatment.

Published by Dr. Loudon Publishing

Dedication

I wish to dedicate this book to my wife, Sylvia.

She has not only helped me but withstood the solitary living room environment, while I was in the computer room writing two cancer books. Also, I wish to dedicate the book to my daughter, Cindy, who was a wonderful help in writing the book.

Unfortunately, Sylvia had a stroke on August 12, 2020. She has been through rehabilitation and is now doing OK. She needs to be in a wheel chair but can walk with help and is doing good.

Lastly, I want to dedicate the book and thank the hundreds of dedicated physicians, biochemists, and researchers who have worked tirelessly to find a cure for cancer.

We are on the verge of curing the dreaded disease.

About the Cover

Dr. Joanna Budwig made some of the greatest cancer discoveries of all time. She was a biochemist who found some severe discrepancies in the red blood cells of cancer patients. She devised a technique to analyze a cancer patient's blood fat metabolism. What she found was a revelation in cancer research. Using her microscope, Dr. Budwig found that the blood in cancer patients had a greenish color. She then found that the color came from blood platelet coagulation (sticky blood), pictured on the cover. Her analysis then led her to discover that almost every cancer patient had coagulated (sticky) blood. This was keeping the red blood cells from carrying oxygen to the body cells. From those findings, she made some revolutionary discoveries. All of this information can be found in chapter 26 of the book.

Another two very important paradigms in curing cancer are the Cell-Sonic Very Intense Pressure Pulse therapy machine, and the Onnetsu 4 in 1 therapy machine (center photo on cover). The Budwig clinic in Spain uses both therapy machines to help cure cancer. Along with the other procedures being used, the Budwig clinic has a very high cure rate for cancer. They plan to open a new clinic in Florida.

These machines also cure many other diseases including kidney stones, wound healing, enlarged prostate, gall stones, rheumatic arthritis, prostate cancer, breast cancer, and many other diseases. These treatment options are very promising. You can learn more about this topic in chapter 27.

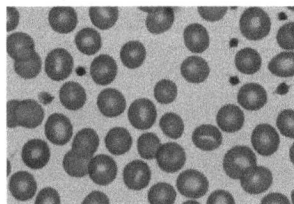

Free Blood

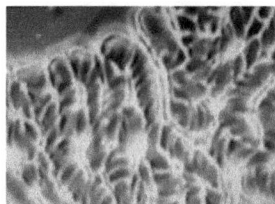

Sticky Blood

Acknowledgments

Had I not met Dr. William Donald Kelley decades ago in Texas, and found out about his cancer treatment, this book would never have been written. Since I have given many lectures on nutrition, I have always been interested in preventing cancer. However, it was not until my brother, Wally, died from lung cancer that I started seriously investigating cancer and its devastating effects. When Dr. Kelley moved within 10 miles of where I grew up and went to high school in Twisp, Washington, I realized that I would find out more about his life and how he started the alternative cancer treatment that cured him and thousands of other people with pancreatic and other cancers.

Shortly afterward, Dr. Nickolas Gonzalez's book, "One Man Alone," was in my possession. It was a powerful inspiration for me. That was the beginning of my serious research on cancer. Dr. Gonzalez has opened many doors with his books and cancer treatment modalities. Further study included information from Drs. Otto Warburg, Linus Pauling, James Beard, Joanna Budwig, Cary Reams, Dr. Brownstein, Dr. Micozzi, the Gerson Clinic, and many others.

I realized that the way cancer treatment was being performed in the U.S. for almost 90 years, cancer treatment was a closed subject, only treating the symptoms of cancer rather than the cure. Thankfully, today, things are changing.

I want to thank several other people who have contributed to their knowledge toward writing this book, Dr. Jim Carlson, Dr. Runar Johnson, Dr. A. F. Beddoe, and Joann Roe. Also, a great thanks to Dr. Wilbur Ricketts, who helped me study those late nights into the mornings while at the University of Washington dental school. He is no longer with us, but often, he referred to pizza as dead food. I did not understand his meaning until many years later. After knowing how cationic, acetic, non-electromagnetic, and low pH foods react in the body, I now realize what Wilbur meant.

Dr. Merle Loudon

Contents

Section I

Information and Discoveries as a Foundation for Preventing and Curing Cancer

Section II

The Parent and Teacher Guide that Explain Nutrition Values in 54 Foods

About the Author

Dr. Merle Loudon is a dentist who has spent 35 years teaching temporal mandibular dysfunction treatment and its relationship with muscles, scoliosis, nutrition, and diet. He graduated from Central Washington University with a degree in organic chemistry and from the University of Washington with a dentistry degree. He has given orthodontics courses, otitis media, temporal mandibular dysfunction, and dysfunctional occlusion related to the cervical vertebrae, nutrition, and cognitive thinking. He has lectured in the US, Canada, and many foreign nations.

In 1980, Dr. Loudon found the fundamental cause of oral malocclusions with his discovery and placement of the tongue positions, nasal versus mouth breathing, and swallowing positions. In 1985, Dr. Loudon found a cure for otitis media with effusion, and its relationship with bite overclosures, the temporal joint, and impingement of the eustachian tube. He has studied, written, and published numerous articles about the relationship and development of occlusions, temporal mandibular joint, otitis media with effusion, oral habits, diet, nutrition, the immune system, and the Eight Rules of Cognitive Thinking.

In 2002, Dr. Loudon studied and started accumulating information on the cause and cure for cancer-related to body electromagnetic diet, electrochemical body cells, and biochemical physiology related to nutrition. He has studied the findings of numerous alternative cancer doctors, naturopaths, and nutritionists. He also studied the treatments used at many alternative cancer clinics, both in Germany and the US.

This book is a compilation of important information relating to the origin of cancer, nutrition, diet, and preventive cancer procedures. It also can be a great help for anyone who has just heard the term. "You have cancer!"

He also studied the cancer treatments used at many alternative cancer clinics in Spain, Germany, Japan, Mexico, and the U.S.

Welcome

Welcome to a journey of exploration into the science of energy, health, nutrition, molecular, and body cell physiology. You will understand how food and nutrition produce the fuel that runs the human body and recognize the foods that keep a person healthy and free from disease.

My book contains information vitally needed to prevent cancer. It explains how cancer patients can improve their health, even if they get conventional cancer treatment with chemotherapy, radiation, and surgery.

The book is divided into two sections. Section I contains information and discoveries that are the foundation for preventing and curing cancer. It also explains the foundation for body nutrition, including how energy and healthy intestinal bacteria are the foundation for excellent health.

God gave us food to produce energy, but he didn't explain what food does or how the body converts and processes food. More importantly, God didn't tell us how food is utilized in the body. This first section of the book will do that.

Section II shows us how the body uses food to produce energy and food that will cause disease. It lists the foods producing good health and the foods that produce bad health.

The second section (Section II) of the book contains information on 54 food choices, good and not good foods, nutrients, and supplements that produce energy in your body, poor health, and disease. These good and not-so-good food choices determine the health of your intestinal bacteria, body cells, blood, and organs.

Section II lists more than 54 of the most common foods, nutrients, and supplement groups. It shows the energy values in food that produce great energy and food that produces little or no energy. The food, nutrient, and supplement groups have been graded on a scale from 10 (great and good energy) down to one (poor or no energy). I also list the magnetic food value, pH, and energy value, plus the nutrition value for keeping good health.

Hippocrates (c. 460 – 370 BC) said, "Let thy food be thy medicine, and let thy medicine be thy food."

This is especially true in preventing or helping to cure cancer.

Disclaimer

All information in this book is for informational purposes only. It should not be interpreted as medical or health treatment.

If any supplement, nutrient, food, remedy, or dosage of supplements are mentioned or written, do not rely on any of this information as medical treatment or medical advice. Any dosages may vary and should be affirmed with your physician or naturopath. Before using any advice, treatment, dosages, or medical content, you should consult with a licensed medical physician or health provider. This book's information is believed to be accurate and sound, based on the best and latest information available. That does not mean that the reader should not consult with a licensed health professional.

Before or when using any information, taking any supplements, remedies, or food mentioned in this book, always check and get your physician's advice or naturopath. If you have any questions or concerns before starting or modifying any cancer treatment, do not rely on this information without your physician's advice or treatment.

Dr. Merle Loudon

Introduction

Thirty-five to forty-five percent of all people in the United States do not eat a healthy diet. The unhealthy effects show up as intestinal toxins, inflammation, leaky bowel syndrome, free radical cell damage, Candida fungus infestations, parasites, and diseases such as diabetes, Crohn's disease, arthritis, high blood pressure, auto-immune conditions, cancer, and other diseases.

Preventing cancer, plus treatments to cure cancer in this book will provide information about how cancer originates, how cancer metastasizes, what you can do to help cure cancer, improving your health, and how cancer prevention relates to eating a healthy diet. Most important, it is a collection of machines, treatments, and ideas to help you prevent and cure cancer. Many of these important procedures are not found anywhere else.

Every year in the US, 1.85 million new cases of cancer are diagnosed. Today, one in three women will have cancer in her lifetime. One in two or three men will have prostate and other cancers. The problem: With tens of billions of dollars spent by cancer patient treatment, donors, and drug company research every year, the true cause and cure of cancer have been stifled by most alternative physicians, for the last 75 years. Chemotherapy, radiation, drugs, and surgery treat the symptoms of cancer, but for many cancers, usually not the cure.

The latest research on cancer treatment has found that some chemo drugs even help create or increase cancer cells by emitting a protein that enhances cancer cell growth but does not kill the stem cells, resulting in the return of cancer. The present methods of treating cancer have not changed much, although, recently, many new treatments, along with combinations of conventional treatment, alternative homeopathic treatments, great new machines, CellSonic Electrohydraulic therapy, 4 in 1 blanket therapy, proton beam therapy, Joanna Budwig's formula, infrared sauna, enzymes, oxygen, removing mercury fillings, and other treatments are helping to cure cancer with fewer side effects.

The basic mechanism and cause for preventing and curing cancer were discovered by the brilliant Nobel-winning genius, Dr. Otto

Warburg, over 95 years ago in 1923. He also laid the foundation for the cure of cancer by proving that cancer cells were multiplying with the process of fermentation, not by oxygenation. Glucose fermentation lets the cancer cells live and multiply without oxygen. Many factors contribute to low oxygen including sugar, refined, processed, and acetic non-electromagnetic foods, lack of exercise, toxins in body cells and organs, bad intestinal bacteria, sugar, omega 6 vegetable oils, parasites, and Candida fungus. Low body oxygen content plus a bad diet, paves the way for toxins, small intestinal inflammation, and free-radical body cell damage to occur, which weakens the mitochondria inside the body cells.

Dr. Otto Warburg, Dr. Linus Pauling, and Dr. Joanna Budwig made some incredible discoveries that are the foundation for treating every cancer patient today. Linus Pauling was a genius. His knowledge in chemistry, biochemistry, physics, theoretical, and applied medicine paved the way for incredible discoveries in treating cancer. Dr. Pauling discovered a polypeptide chain formed with amino acids, that would coil into a helix structure he called "the alpha helix." The alpha helix carbon molecule paved the way for many food formulas that are still used today in treating cancer. He would have gotten another Nobel prize for his discovery, but two other scientists sent their work ahead of Dr. Pauling when he was delayed in getting to England to present his findings.

Dr. Joanna Budwig, a biochemist, and researcher followed up on Dr. Pauling's alpha helix discovery by finding a double bond helix formula that would unravel sticky blood. She found that most cancer patients produced a substance called homocysteine, a substance in the blood that caused coagulation of the red blood platelets (sticky blood). That led her to the cottage cheese, flaxseed oil, quark, and crushed flaxseed formula to help unravel the sticky blood. Cancer cells love an acetic body, plus low oxygen levels from sugared foods, refined and processed carbohydrates, refined, acetic, non-electromagnetic foods, preservatives, and lack of oxygen. Increased toxins in body cells, organs plus bad intestinal bacteria, pave the way for dangerous intestinal inflammation, leaky gut, free radical body cell damage, lactic acid buildup, cell oxygen suffocation, fermentation, and then cancer cell metabolism. In the years since Dr. Warburg's discovery, the FDA, U.S. drug companies, and the government have choked off attempts to use homeopathic and alternative natural therapies for preventing and curing cancer. The proof is the lack of diet information by physicians and the lack of GMO labels on our food packages. Most physicians use only drugs, radiation, surgery, and chemo products from drug companies to cure cancer. They skip informing the patient about diet, exercise, coffee enemas, detoxification, Candida fungus, and parasite elimination, plus the use of pancreatic enzymes. The government also allows Monsanto's unhealthy food products to stay on the market, with government laws that keep labels from being put on Monsanto's GMO foods.

The worst crimes of all are the unsubstantiated mysterious deaths of 77 alternative cancer doctors and functional health physicians. Many deaths (between 2015 and 2019) from murders and supposed suicides have not been solved. One of these deaths involved a very dedicated and wonderful alternative cancer physician, Dr. Nicholas Gonzalez. In the meantime, not one reported mysterious death of the cancer oncologists who use chemo, surgery, or radiation treatment has occurred.

The FDA, drug companies, and cancer physicians have raked in about 180 to 200 billion dollars per year on cancer treatment. Although they have saved many people's lives, think of all the millions of people, many of whom may have been your relatives and friends, who have died with the regular oncologist's 55-percent-average five-year success rate with their cancer treatment. Most oncologists will not mention the great use of a special cancer diet, plus adding alternative cancer treatment, with new electrical impulse machines, oxygen, coffee enemas, IV vitamin C, IV mistletoe, intestinal cleansing, detoxification, and pancreatic enzymes.

Many European and Far Eastern physicians, using alternative cancer treatments, are getting a 75 percent to 85 percent cancer cure success rate. Many patients are living for more years than five. In the US, the overall average success rate other than proton therapy for all cancer patients living more than five years is about 55 percent, and less for some cancers. Recently, there have been improvements in some types of cancer treatment, but much more is needed.

One of the more recent cancer treatments is a newer therapy machine that is being used with remarkable success in helping to cure many types of cancer. Dr. Joanna Budwig's cancer clinic in Spain has introduced two new machines that are available in Spain.

One machine is called; The CellSonic Electrohydraulic therapy machine. Cancer cells have a weakened electric charge (ionic and cationic electrical impulses). The CellSonic therapy machine switches the polarity, increases the cell electrical impulses, and changes the polarity of the cancer cells (and also other disease cells), from a disease molecular alignment to a correct body cell alignment. It works with a process of shockwaves that provoke cancer cells. The waves are generated with electric voltages which are directed by a handheld pointer, into the cancer area. The remarkable thing about the CellSonic therapy machine is that it also can treat many other diseases and complications including wound healing, enlarged prostates, many cancers, gall stones, kidney stones, stenosis, avascular necrosis, and many other conditions. All of these treatments for cancer and many diseases are noninvasive and do not require much time. The CellSonic machine can also be used with chemo, radiation, and chemo drugs, but THE PATIENT needs to WAIT TWO TO FOUR WEEKS to have the CellSonic treatments. The treatments are a lot less expensive than chemo, radiation, surgery, or drugs. Another new machine is the "4 in 1 blanket." It has had some remarkable results so far.

Many physicians still say that cancer is from a genetic trait, and that genetic mutation is the precursor to cancer. However, recent research has shown that for almost all cases, it is not the root cause.

Cancer physicians in many foreign countries have had great success in treating patients who live for five years or more. For 75 percent to 85 percent of their patients, the cancer is cured.

How have these cancer physicians been so successful? By using many alternative cancer treatments including CellSonic electrohydraulic therapy, IV vitamin C and mistletoe, Joanna Budwig's formula, coffee enemas, nitric oxide supplements, pure raw vegetables, and vegetable juices, sunshine, hot baths, and saunas. Also by restricting their diet by eliminating processed and refined foods, red meat, Omega 6 oils on the grocery shelf, increasing their oxygen intake by giving them a live food diet, vegetable juices, neutral or alkaline pH foods, electromagnetic, oxygen-rich energy foods, probiotics, fermented foods, supplements that raise and help increase blood oxygen, enzymes, creating free-flowing red blood cells, exercise, liver and gall bladder detoxification that creates oxygen cell metabolism at the cellular level, and eliminating the toxins inside of the intestines, which create a barrier to absorption of the enzymes and nutrients. Also by removing all mercury fillings.

With many new treatments, cell destruction doses of chemo and radiation, destroy less regular cancer and stem cells. This does not destroy as much of the people's good cells and immune system.

Section I

**Information and Discoveries as a Foundation
for Preventing and Curing Cancer.**

1

The Greatest Medical Hoax in U.S. History

A person who lives in the U.S. doesn't hear much about the medical system and how pharmaceutical companies, the FDA, and even the government in certain areas, such as GMOs, control it.

Political corruption is everywhere. The political corruption in the United States is so widespread that it extends right up to the steps of the White House. It has invaded our government in a powerful destructive way. Crooked politicians and billionaires, large mega-corporations, the media, CIA, FBI, FDA, drug companies, and foreign countries that are not our friends control most political corruption in the U.S. This corruption creates an immense disaster for our freedoms, liberty, laws, children, grandchildren, and even poor people who are just trying to survive.

Webster's Dictionary describes corruption as "pervasive or deterioration of moral principles, attaining treason or felony, deprivation, adulteration, taint, bribery, to destroy, bribe, contaminate, pervert, make or become corrupt." Treason is defined as 1. Violation of the allegiance owed to one's sovereign state and/or betrayal of the United States constitution. 2. Any betraying, treachery, breach of faith, or betrayal of trust in the constitution.

The formula for corruption is to use pressure for blackmail, infiltrate companies or nations for technical information, induce population control, people control, use U.S. taxpayers' money and leverage it for personal, family greed, money or seduce people for money, and information. Politicians create massive multi-billion military and government contracts and receive a kickback behind the back for a politician's signature and/or give secrets to foreign countries for money. These actions deprive companies that will enhance health and welfare from legally operating, while politicians are making laws that are not truthful in their meaning and objectives, etc. Much of this corruption edges up to the act of treason.

1

Have you ever wondered why American citizens in the U.S. pay four to five times more for medical treatment than people in all other countries? What is the reason for our high medical costs, and when did this situation and Medical hoax begin? Why don't we have a definite cure for many diseases, including cancer, diabetes, and high blood pressure? Where does all the money for medical treatment go? How did Big Pharma end up being our biggest medical treatment system? These questions and more need many answers and solutions, We need to solve the problems and change the most expensive medical system in the world.

There is no doubt that we all need physicians and associates to treat our many ills and diseases. They do an excellent job for most of our life-saving treatment and medical ills. But something has gone wrong with many medical treatments and drugs that are being given today. This is especially true in the treatment of cancer. In the shadows a long time ago, a certain millionaire connived to develop and control our U.S. medical system. From the very beginning, he developed a plan to start a system that ended up being big Pharma, and the control of our medical system, colleges, drug companies, and doctors.

The following is hard to believe. Before 1878 most medical treatments in the U.S. were from plant-based and homeopathic medicine. Almost all countries today use diet recommendations, homeopathic treatment, cannaboid medications, plus modern treatments and machines. They not only surpass the U.S. in successful cures of cancer, diabetes, high blood pressure, and other diseases but have four to five times less cost for the patient.

We can trace the beginnings of Big Pharma to John D Rockefeller in 1878. He controlled a vast oil empire and made millions of dollars with over 80 percent of the oil business. Cars were just invented and the use of oil was just beginning. But his grandiose ideas in medicine and medical treatment came about in 1897 when the discovery of aspirin was made by Felix Hoffman, a German scientist. Rockefeller knew that a new medical frontier opened up with the use of petrochemicals. He visualized that petrochemicals could be the foundation for medicine including aspirin, penicillin, and other treatment drugs.

Rockefeller realized that to expand his medical empire, he would have to change the plant-based homeopathic medicine to a petrochemical medicine domination. This would be no small task.

First, he established the Rockefeller Institute for Medical Research. His leader, Fredrick Gates, in 1901, was influenced by a new book, "Principles and Practice of Medicine," written by Sir William Osler. Osler was an early pioneer of "Eugenics", the study of hereditary improvement by genetic control. What is interesting about this is that C.C. Little, a eugenics follower, and early president of the American Cancer Society, became the founding member of the Birth Control League, which eventually became known as "Planned Parenthood."

In 1913, Rockefeller, his son, and Fredrick Gates joined in a new project. The goal was to justify the modernization, streamlining, and consolidation of medical teaching in medical schools and hospitals. This effort forced out most of the teaching for plant-based homeopathic medicine. This was a greedy, control effort that then changed the course of medicine in the United States. Many homeopathic schools were closed, many hospitals had to change their direction from plant-based treatments. Some doctors were even jailed. This was the beginning of a new era, "a pill for every ill."

After 1913, all medical schools and hospitals, to receive Rockefeller grants and money, were directed to teach and do research in the directed medical areas where these newly discovered drugs could be patented and sold in the many drug outlets within the Rockefeller empire. This included Squibb, which, at the time, was a wholly-owned Rockefeller business. New, great helpful medicines, techniques, and medical machines that were not sanctioned by the FDA were denied by the FDA and drug companies. The practice is still going on today. Many great treatments and machines that are being used to cure cancer in other countries are being restricted for use in the U.S.

In 1938, the discovery of penicillin boosted Rockefeller's fortunes. During world war II, Big Pharma was well established and bringing in high profits. They were filtering money to the FDA, lobbyists, drug companies, and even cancer doctors. Over the past many years, big pharma has entrenched itself into the ropes of the government, FDA, lobbyists, drug companies, and doctors. Also, many of the smaller drug companies were bought out by the larger firms. Researchers say more than 50 percent of all Americans are over medicated. The Rockefeller dream has cost the U.S. patients millions of dollars. It has increased the insurance company's medical charges and profits of millions of dollars. Now, medical treatments and drugs cost American patients over 500 billion dollars a year, 200 billion for cancer alone. The cure rate for cancer in the U.S., on average, is about 55 percent for people living over 5 years. In some types of cancer, it is much higher.

My brother Jim was diagnosed with lymphoma. His medical insurance company paid out about $13,000.00 per month for chemotherapy. Over 4 years of treatment, the insurance costs were over $500,000.00. The treatment did not cure his lymphoma but subdued and retarded it over that time.

But there is some hope. New research, artificial intelligence, electric pulse machines like the VIPP therapy machine, and the Onestsu 4 in 1 blanket, both used by the Budwig cancer clinic are helping to cure cancer. Plant-based and homeopathic medicines and cannabinoids have begun to increase many new treatment modalities, plus alternative functional medicine is on the rise. Maybe we will see some great changes soon.

Most of the corruption in this country is because there are two opposing sets of principles. They are involved with medical treatment control, the media, pharmaceutical drugs, the billionaires, the politicians, large mega-companies, some law agencies, the lobbyists, the conservatives, and the liberals. Until we get back to the same set of rules set out by the constitution, we will have no just law, mob violence, crooked elections, breach of laws, anarchy, a one-world agenda, violence, extreme corruption, even treason, and a downhill spiral into oblivion.

Many things need to be changed soon. If we do not have the truth, constitutional laws, elimination of the deep state, honest elections, and stop the corruption and treason we will be left with the crumbs, and then it will be too late. We are reaching the boiling point.

2

The Soil: Source of Energy, Health and Oxygen

The relationship of energy and oxygen to body health involves the relationship with the dynamics and minerals in the soil. There are some very important correlations between the soil and the many biological processes that are created in the human body. To understand this, you have to take a look at the nutrients and minerals in the soil and how it produces energy in a person's body.

The soil has many minerals. More than sixty-five minerals are needed for the metabolism of our body cells and organs. Most of these minerals, especially calcium, magnesium, zinc, phosphate, selenium, potassium, and other minor minerals, are picked up from the roots of plants. The minerals are consumed, transferred, and assimilated, not only in humans but also into the bodies of all animals, birds, bacteria, parasites, and some viruses. Vital raw nutrients such as fiber, amino acids, enzymes, and vitamins from these trees, plants, and minerals are all vitally needed to produce electromagnetic energy in the body. Electromagnetic energy in body molecules is what creates and maintains the health of a person.

To understand energy, a person needs to know the difference between an anion and a cation. Anion atoms or cation atoms are found in every cell and molecule of plants, trees, animals, birds, fish, and other living organisms. They end up making the anionic and cationic atoms, molecules, body cells, and organs that are produced in your body. Most anions and cations used in the body come from live plants, minerals, trees, seeds, nuts, essential oils, seafood, and fish products. These foods produce and make energy in the body from the roots and nutrients of the living trees, plants, animals, and other organisms. These foods also make up the vitamins, enzymes, amino acids, RNA, DNA, and other essential elements in a person's body cells.

The anion and cation atoms have opposite charges generated by the rotations of the electrons in the atoms. To simplify the chemistry, the anions have electrons that rotate in a clockwise direction and have a negative charge. Being a negatively charged atom, an anion atom has more electrons than neutrons. Cations have almost the same nucleus but have electrons that rotate counterclockwise in the outer orbit. They are positively charged and have fewer electrons than protons.

Why is this so important? Because these two different types of atoms, with opposite moving electrons, create energy. They create the resistance (energy) that is in our molecules and cells. The energy from anions and cations is brought about by transferring the minerals, protein, essential oils, seeds, and plant nutrients into the human bodies to produce the enzymes, vitamins, amino acids, and other constituents needed in the blood, body organs, immune system, and other body cells. Cations and anions are both needed to create energy in our bodies. If there is no potential energy, no energy is produced.

Dr. Carey Reams states that most foods that are eaten are cationic. As they enter the stomach and small intestine, the anionic enzymes create anionic (alkaline) cells, if the foods are electromagnetic. If the foods are non-electromagnetic, they are not changed to electromagnetic, ionic cells. Most of the electromagnetic foods, raw fresh vegetables, fruits, melons, seeds, nuts, leaves, roots, essential oils, proteins, supplements, and other nutrients consumed produce the energy that is created in your body. Most of the non-electromagnetic cationic foods, sugars, oils on the grocery shelf, GMO foods, refined and processed foods that you consume can become acidic, produce little or no energy, and do just the opposite. They create damaging elements that create toxins, harm your intestinal bacteria, body, cells, and organs. Too much cationic, non-electromagnetic food causes acidity, toxins, inflammation, leaky gut, free radical body cells, and disease.

The electromagnetic measure of this energy (resistance) is called pH. It can be measured by a product called pHydrion litmus paper. Hydrion litmus paper strips can be purchased online, at Amazon, or in some health food stores.

A good acid/alkaline measurement of body pH can be done by measuring the blood and saliva. This is done with Hydrion litmus paper, inserted in the liquids. The optimum, neutral, efficient body cell (urine and saliva) pH range is 6.2 to 6.8. Lower ranges (urine and saliva 6.1 and lower), create an acidic range. The lower the acidic range from 6.2, the more damaging it can be to body health. A higher alkaline range from normal (urine and saliva 6.8), is also damaging, but not as severe as an acidic range. This very important measurement is related to your blood (7.4 pH), organs, (7.4 pH), and body cells.

With a good electromagnetic diet, the blood and body cell pH can be kept at 7.4. This helps create the proper cell pH, blood pH, and heart rhythm.. Keeping a neutral body cell, blood, urine, and saliva pH is very helpful, and essential for good health. The heart utilizes a neutral pH and body calcium to create a steady rhythm. When the body cell and blood pH get critically low, the blood calls out in the blood for body calcium to maintain a constant rhythm. The calcium then comes from calcium in the bone and cartilage cells.

With good food choices (raw fresh vegetables, fruits, berries, melons, nuts, leaves, essential oils, and proteins) the body produces more anions than cations. That is healthy and good. In the second section of this book, the foods are rated according to the pH, nutrition, and energy that they produce. Almost always, the more energy a food produces, the more healthful it is. Raw, fresh, anionic foods provide great energy benefits for people's health, oxygen metabolism, and suppression of the disease. High energy produces less inflammation and free radical molecules in your cells. It also creates less arthritis, lower blood pressure, less heart disease, fewer colds, other diseases, and less Candida albicans fungus in your intestines. This correlates with a healthier gut, better digestion, a better immune system, and many other wonderful health benefits.

3

Electromagnetic Body Energy

Most people do not realize that electromagnetic voltage (pH or acid/alkaline balance) is the motor that runs our energy produced in our blood cells, body cells, and body organs. It is easy for people to shop in the grocery store to buy foods that have little or no electromagnetic (energy) value. Examples are processed foods, sugar, sugar products, preservatives, and especially all vegetable oils found on the grocery shelf, except extra virgin olive oil. Even extra virgin olive oil, if it is not in a dark container, or not kept in the refrigerator, can become an omega 6 oil, a partially or completely non-electromagnetic or "dead" oil.

Some non-electromagnetic (cationic) foods in small amounts may not harm your health, including foods with some carbohydrates, minerals, and fiber. However, continued moderate to heavy consumption of these cationic "dead" non-electromagnetic foods causes body cell acidity and negative changes to your energy. They also create toxins, an inflammatory intestinal lining, leaky gut (holes in the small intestine), toxin invasion into the blood, and radical body cell changes to your blood, body cells, organs, digestive bacteria, digestive and immune system.

A non-electromagnetic, acidic diet will create chronic inflammation and radical body cell damage. It will cause many changes including the creation of an acetic (cationic) body that depletes the good bacteria in your small intestine. This diet causes an increase in gut toxins, gut inflammation, intestinal Candida fungus, bad bacteria, and parasite population. The chronic acidic diet can increase the bad bacteria, candida, and change the intestinal flora. When bad bacteria overcome the good bacteria in the small intestine, they can produce toxins, which cause inflammation of the small intestinal wall. This causes a leaky gut. Toxins, parasite larvae, bad bacteria, and other bad hombre get into the blood. This is the start of a disease state. These products cause radical cell damage and even damage the DNA and RNA in the mitochondria. It is now known that increased bad bacteria, parasites, toxins, candida

8

fungus, plus an acetic body, is associated with the start and spread of cancer in many individuals.

Fresh, cold, raw polyunsaturated plant and fish oils, raw live plant food, plus their derivatives, seeds, or food made from them, create an anionic electromagnetic environment that increases the vitality and electromagnetic energy in your body. These raw oils and foods create healthier blood, body cells, and the immune system. Anionic alkaline diets will also crowd out the bad bacteria and candida fungus in your intestines. It is hard to believe, but about 80 percent of your immune system is in your intestines when mostly healthy bacteria are present. These healthy bacteria are responsible for keeping your body cells, organs, red blood cells, and white blood cells (immune system) healthy, plus helping them operate to optimum levels.

If good intestinal bacteria are not present, bad bacteria, candida, and bad bacteria parasites can take over the premises. The toxins and inflammation get into the blood via leaky gut (small holes in the intestine). Disease states start to creep in. Blood starts to become sticky and unhealthy. Body cell changes, radical cell damage, blood, intestinal and organ diseases, plus autoimmune diseases, begin their nasty journey into your body cells and joints.

About one million people in the United States die from cancer every year. The statement sometimes used by oncologists is that the body's genes cause cancer. This is not true. Cancer producing non-electromagnetic substances in your blood, body cells, and organs cause mitochondrial changes in the cell DNA and RNA. These chemical changes, or "hits," cause cancer cells to form.

Substances such as refined foods, processed foods, sugar, sugar products, all vegetable oils (not refrigerated) sold on the grocery shelves, nitrates, body cosmetics, chemicals, preservatives, air pollution, chemotherapy drugs, metals, candida Albicans fungus, body parasites, and other non-electromagnetic toxins produce foods and substances that get into your blood. These poisonous substances, plus stress and worry, are the cause of diseases and cancer.

The blood, then, can be the carrier of toxins and non-electromagnetic substances that travel to all parts of your body. That means the pH (acid/alkaline balance) and blood constituents determine your body's cell health, cell division, and environment. The blood delivers oxygen and healthy substances and/or toxins, bad bacteria, and candida, the latter being the cause of diseases. The blood is a delivery and waste removal system. It nurses cells and even has a communication system with the brain and gut biome (flora). It carries oxygen, nourishment, minerals, enzymes, vitamins, and other body products. But it can also carry bad bacteria, candida fungus, viruses, parasite larvae, etc.

Blood composition includes new forming blood, nutrients in the blood, white blood cells, and oxygen. But on the other hand, it can carry inflammatory substances, toxins, bad bacteria, parasites, and other nonessential toxic products, delivered to your body cells and organs

4

The Importance of Anions, Cations, and pH

In the last chapter we discussed anions and cations. But how do anions and cations relate to our food? Anionic foods are raw, fresh, or slightly cooked vegetables, white meat, eggs, raw nuts, berries, fermented food, raw milk and polyunsaturated raw omega-3 oils. Anionic (alkaline) foods should be the biggest part of a person's diet if they want to stay healthy and prevent diseases, including cancer. Examples of cationic foods are sugars, sugar products, carbohydrates, refined and processed foods, omega-6 vegetable oils, and all oils sold on the grocery shelf except extra virgin olive oil. To stay healthy, people need to eat much more anionic, raw, or slightly cooked foods, minerals, nutrients and supplements than they eat cationic foods. Ionic foods should be the biggest part of a person's diet if they want to stay healthy and prevent diseases, including cancer.

If a person eats more cationic foods than ionic foods, the toxins and pH balance will get out of whack. The person's body will become usually more acetic (low pH) or sometimes more alkaline (high pH). Inflammation and free-radical cell damage then occurs, causing diseases to wander and thrive in the body. Dr. Carey Reams (1982) has stated that checking your pH or acid-base balance is one of the most important daily measurements for diagnosing human health and illness. Checking your saliva and urine pH readings every morning and night with hydrion litmus paper before brushing your teeth may be one of the wisest things you can do for your health. The reason is that knowing your pH (acid-base) balance is a check for diagnosing health problems before they occur. You can correct the majority of health problems with your diet. Dr. Reams said that preventing and correcting these acetic-alkaline medical problems and pH balance with your diet can begin long before you need medication for the medical problems.

Most Americans do not even know what pH readings are and what they measure in a person's body. Your body is 70 percent water, two parts hydrogen and one part oxygen. The pH measurement shows your body's acid-alkaline balance. By using a test of body liquids (urine and saliva), you are finding the hydrogen ion potential, or whether your body is acid, alkaline or neutral. This is very important, and involves your diet, health, and wellness.

pH is measured on a scale of 1 (very acidic) to 14 (very alkaline). The middle pH range (6.2 to 6.8) is where the body operates in a healthful, disease free state. When the pH gets acidic or alkaline the body blood, cells, organs and intestinal bacteria get out of balance creating disease states. The more acidic or alkaline (lower or higher pH range) the body gets, the more of an increase in body cell inflammation and free-radical cell damage. When these extreme ranges are diagnosed, your diet usually is the cause. Chronic inflammation, leaky gut and free-radical cell damage from an acetic diet can result in diseases such as arthritis, Crohn's disease, high blood pressure, heart disease, diabetes, asthma, leukocytosis, candida infestation, cancer, and other diseases. Also very important is that a low (acetic) pH will help change the good bacteria in your intestines to bad bacteria, candida fungus, and possibly parasites.

The majority of people in the US eat a cationic diet, and are pH-acidic. Why is this important? Because their body fluids (pH) are showing that the diet they are eating is not an electromagnetic, anionic, live-food, raw vegetable, nut, and omega-3 oil diet. The non-electromagnetic, mostly low pH foods they are eating are causing an acid disease producing state. This is why there is so much obesity, leaky gut, Crohn's disease, leukocytosis, parasites, arthritis, diabetes, heart disease, candida fungus, cancer, and many other diseases.

The pH of the saliva and urine indicates the balance of the fluids that you are excreting. If the pH shows low acid, usually more alkaline foods are needed to raise the pH to a healthy 6.2 to 6.8 pH range. Low acetic pH shows that your alkaline reserves are diminished, and need replenished. The narrow healthy middle pH range, 6.2 to 6.8 (green pH paper) and in the optimum body pH range, shows that the person is eating a diet of high electromagnetic foods.

Sugar, excess carbs, refined foods, many processed foods, red meat and all non electromagnetic "dead" vegetable oils (except extra virgin olive oil) on the grocery shelf are the worst acetic and disease producing foods.

Section Two of this book lists most of the common foods, nutrients and supplements that most people eat. They are listed according to the electromagnetic range, pH, and nutrition rating. These ratings will tell you if the foods you are buying at the grocery store and eating are a healthy electromagnetic or unhealthy food.

How to Restore an Unhealthy pH:

If you are acidic, there are several things you can eat to raise an unhealthy, acidic pH. One of the best food combinations that can help raise and maintain neutral pH is one that Dr. Johanna Budwig uses for her cancer treatment patients. It is cottage cheese, crushed flaxseeds, and flaxseed oil with added quark. It can be eaten every day, or a minimum of four to seven times weekly. You can add a few berries, pineapple, or pieces of fruit for taste. This combination helps neutralize the pH and the homocysteine (sticky clotting factor) in your blood, which can occur when pH is acidic. The author has found that if the urine and saliva pH at night is acetic, the Budwig combination before bedtime is a great food to raise the pH during the night. Ice cream and sweet desserts will always lower the pH, and are not recommended before bedtime.

If your urine pH is acidic, calcium, vitamin D3, magnesium, potassium, turmeric and L-arginine may help to raise it. Also helpful are raw green vegetable drinks, lemon juice, raw green vegetables, cottage cheese, kefir, flaxseed oil, and ground chia and flaxseeds.

If your saliva pH at night is acidic, polyunsaturated oils (omega-3), lemon juice (two to three tablespoons in water), at night and in the early morning will help. Check your pH before brushing. If saliva pH is acidic, you can also use these supplements: turmeric, L-arginine, Ginkgo biloba, and garlic capsules.

Being too alkaline can also be a factor in causing disease, but it is not as critical as being acidic. If you find your pH is alkaline in the morning or evening, it is wise to bring the pH down to the neutral pH level. When your body is alkaline, you can take ground psyllium husks, flaxseed, cucumber, fish, or northern seed oils (in capsules), or any other fiber that you get with fresh vegetables (7 to 11 different ones a day) ; also enzymes (wobenzym-N with every meal), 2000 mg. vitamin C a day, cottage cheese, apples, pears, grapes, and watermelons.

Raising the pH in the Evening

It is wise not to eat any red meat, sugar or sugar products, ice cream, cereal, etc., after 5:00 p.m. The best and most helpful way to raise your pH before bedtime is the use of cottage cheese, quark and flaxseed oil, Udo's Choice, or raw northern seed oils. Another way is to put two to three tablespoons of lemon juice in a glass of water and drink it before going to bed.

You can obtain hydrion litmus paper strips online or in most health food stores. Buy strips that have a range of 5.0 to 8.0. For easy access you should keep them on your bathroom counter next to your toilet. Check your saliva and urine when you arise in the morning, and before brushing your teeth at night.

In review, if you are very serious about staying healthy and disease-free, you need to be able to check for acidity of your body cells. 40 to 50 percent of all Americans are chronically over-acidic. The only way I know to monitor your pH is with hydrion litmus paper strips. I urge you to consider obtaining a pH (roll) system. Section two of this book will explain how to raise your body pH and/or keep a neutral pH.

Keeping a neutral pH (6.4 to 6.4) is the indication that your body acid/base balance is running on all six cylinders. When you stay pH balanced (6.4 – 6.8) your chances of staying healthy, disease-free, and cancer-free are greatly enhanced. There are numerous research articles showing that cancer thrives in an acidic, cationic, and low oxygen environment. In contrast, a neutral or slightly alkaline body cell environment (pH 6.4 to 7.0) and 7.4 pH blood help to deter or combat and eliminate diseases, including cancer cells. Alkaline, anionic foods raise the electromagnetic energy in blood, organs and body cells, keeping a healthy body and immune system.

The more acidic a person's diet, the less oxygen that is able to get into your blood and body cells. This is just what cancer cells like and thrive in. That is why most alternative cancer treatment centers do all that they can to provide as much oxygen and alkaline foods as possible for their cancer patients.

Johanna Budwig was the first biochemist to recognize that certain foods provided a double-helix-bond carbon molecule, which, in certain foods, unwound sticky (homocysteine) blood. Every day, she prescribed for her cancer patients a mixture of cottage cheese, flaxseed oil, flaxseeds ground in a coffee grinder, and quark. This mixture separated the red blood cells which were clumped together, and increased the flow of oxygen to the body cells. This is very important in cancer treatment.

Oxygen therapy is also very critical in cancer treatment. This is also why many cancer therapists use hyperbaric oxygen, IV vitamin C, raw fresh vegetable and fruit juices, exercise, and oxygen producing supplements such as L-arginine, turmeric, Ginkgo biloba, cesium, DMSO, resveratrol, and other oxygen-producing nitric oxide supplements. They are used to increase the oxygen and raise the pH in the body. Acidic, cationic diets, especially those that include sugars, omega-6 vegetable oils, and red meat, will also restrict the body cell membranes from exchanging oxygen, nutrients and minerals into the cells, and restrict the CO_2, toxins and waste from getting out of the cells. The more acidic the diet, the more restricted the body cell membranes become, which causes them to get weaker. The weaker the body cells, the easier cancer will creep in. Weak cells help to sustain more inflammation, free-radical cell damage, changes in the DNA, and the chance of cancer, and they can make it more difficult to eliminate cancer cells.

If a person is serious about body pH, they will check their urine and saliva morning and night. It is best to check the pH before eating anything or brushing the teeth. A person will find that an alkaline diet is one of the best ways to prevent inflammation, radical body cell and organ damage. It is also the secret to more energy, less fatigue, and in most cases, a longer life. When your diet becomes more neutral and optimum (pH of 6.4 to 7.0 routinely), the cell wall permeability increases. The O2, minerals and nutrients can enter the cells effortlessly, and the CO_2, wastes, and toxins get out easily. Oxygen will be in a healthy range, and the blood cells will be separated and carry a sufficient amount of oxygen. This may take some time, as a person's body may not reflect the change immediately after starting a more alkaline diet. If at first you can't seem to neutralize your pH, stay on the alkalizing diet, and normally your metabolism will change.

There are some other things that also help in the quest for a normal-pH electromagnetic cell health.

Some of these things are:

1. Checking calcium intake. Calcium is a very important alkalizing mineral. Some calcium tablets are much better than others. Coral calcium, calcium orotate, calcium lactate, and canned sardines and herring are all very good calcium. Tums® and some other forms of calcium are not assimilated as well by the body, and are not as effective as others. Remember, magnesium is needed to assimilate calcium in the body. It should be a daily requirement.

2. Two or three glasses of raw, fresh vegetable juice with lemon juice is one of the best foods for preventing as well as treating cancer. It is used by the Gerson clinic. Gerson believed that for making the juice, a person should use 7 to 11 different raw vegetables and fruits, with lemons. This is always a great food, whether you want to prevent cancer or are being treated with cancer. It has been recorded that a cancer patient ate and drank nothing but eight to ten glasses of vegetable and fruit juice every day. In 6 months, all signs of his cancer were gone. It is usually not used as a single treatment, but with other modalities as well.

3. Alkaline water is also being used by some practitioners. It is hard to find the right percentage, and should only be used if percentages are known.

4. Lemon juice is one of the best ways to raise the body cell pH. Two to three tablespoons of pure fresh squeezed lemon juice in a small glass of water before going to bed, and also first thing in the morning, will really be a boost in raising your pH. Lemon juice stimulates the pancreas to produce alkalizing enzymes. Lemons help raise the pH. Dr. Cary

Reams (1982) says that only fresh squeezed lemons should be used, along with distilled water.

5. Water is also one of the most important things to maintain a neutral pH. The pH of good water is 7.4. Water is a neutralizer for the body. It not only helps excrete wastes from the body, but helps to maintain continued neutral pH readings. It also helps maintain the blood pH of 7.4, which is critical. Distilled water is the more pure, and especially the best for preventing cancer and for cancer patients.

Be sure that you refrain from drinking water in plastic bottles. Plastic bottles contain bisphenol-A (BPA), a hormone related to estrogen. Plastic is causing men to get way too much estrogen. That needs to be balanced with testosterone. Testosterone is now one of the most used supplements sold to men in the US.

There has been some research on BLA elixir. BLA elixir blocks lactic acid removal from cancer cells. The result is apoptosis, or death of the cancer cells. More needs to be learned about this procedure. Remember that the best way to prevent cancer and to eradicate cancer is to keep a neutral pH of 6.4–7.0. We hope that your prevention or treatment of cancer includes the use of pH strips.

5

Dr. Otto Warburg: The Man Who Found the Cause of Cancer

Dr. Otto Warburg was a biochemist and physiologist. He won a Nobel Prize in 1931 for his many discoveries, and for finding the root cause of cancer. Actually, he found the route (road) that a normal body cell takes to become a cancer cell. His discoveries were instrumental from a biochemical standpoint, cell metabolism, cell morphology, and most of all, a route for curing cancer.

His very important findings were that the root cause of cancer is from a body-cell oxygen deficiency, coupled with a deficiency of cell alkalinity (low pH), and fermentation of body and cancer cells by glycolysis, which was an enormous discovery.

Normal blood and body cells require oxygen. The body gets its oxygen from the lungs and from the anionic (live) foods a person eats. He discovered that too much acidic (high cationic, low pH) foods in the body, created by foods such as sugar, bad vegetable oils, alcohol, red meat, and many other low-pH foods, creates acidosis and a lack of oxygen to the blood and body cells. The diagram below will show Dr. Warburg's route from a normal body or blood cell to a cancer cell.

Poor diet, not enough anionic foods (low pH)	→	Increased cell acidy	→	Reduced O2 levels in blood & body cells	→	Normal cells cannot convert enough O2

Mitochondria mutation changes normal cells to Cancer cells	←	Destruction of RNA and DNA (changes in amino acids)	←	Lactic acid lowers cell pH (more acidity), cells become damaged	←	Excess lactic acid is produced creating fermentation

Cancer cells begin to multiply (blood becomes sticky) cannot carry oxygen to body cells	→	Creates the anaerobic conditions that cancer cells love

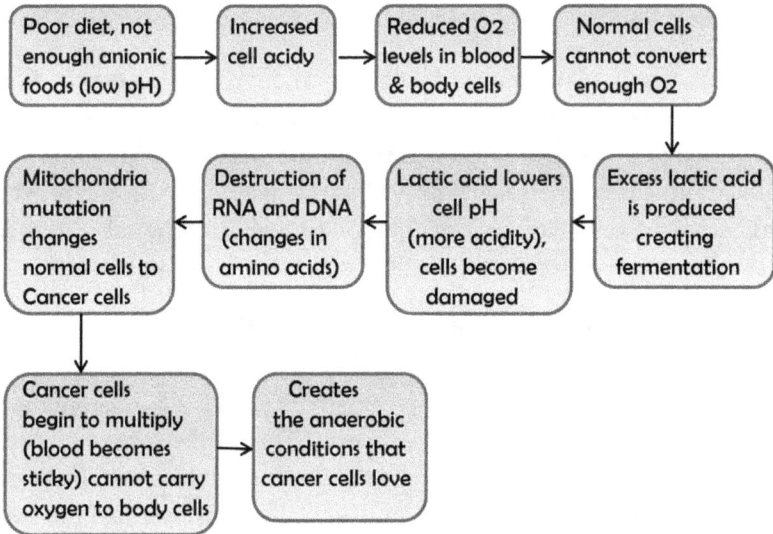

Research has shown that Candida albicans fungus is intertwined
with cancer cells 80 percent of the time.

Further research by Dr. Warburg (2015c) showed that once a person has cancer, the cancer cells will not live in an alkaline pH of 7.4 or higher. He also showed that high concentrations of oxygen slowed and stopped cancer cells.

The ironic part of Dr. Warburg's discoveries is that the drug companies, FDA and medical doctors have had almost 90 years to develop alternative ways to cure cancer. Instead, they have spent billions of dollars (especially the FDA and drug companies) finding expensive chemo drugs and radiation treatments, when that money could have gone into curing cancer with alternative methods, which are used in Europe, but are now just beginning to come out in the US. Instead, the medical and drug establishment elected to create a money-making treatment, costing people 180 to 200 billion dollars per year. After showing that lack of body cell oxygen causes a fermentation of sugar and cancer metabolism, Dr. Warburg showed the very critical consequences of oxygen deprivation. He proved that lack of body cell oxygen triggers the body cells to start using glucose to provide the oxygen. They become partially anaerobic. This causes an impaired oxygen environment, which damages the chemical makeup of mitochondria inside the cells. The

DNA then gets chemically changed, which switches regular body cells to cancer cells.

Other scientists later proved that after prolonged oxygen deprivation, the body cell's mitochondria and DNA could became abnormal. They confirmed this was the switch that turns on cancer cell origination and replication. Their experiments proved that cancer cells can thrive with little or no oxygen, plus use fermentation to replicate. They also showed that excessive oxygen therapy could also reverse this process.

The experiments of Dr. Warburg and other scientists found the root cause of cancer. More importantly, they showed that in replicating, cancer cells produced incredibly excessive amounts of inflammation, free-radical cell damage, and waste toxins. This weakens the body cell system, including the blood, cells, organs, immune system, and intestinal bacteria. More importantly, these life-sucking toxins overload the liver and coat the intestines with a crust-like substance that causes a barrier and does not allow nutrients, enzymes, vitamins, amino acids, and supplements to get into the bloodstream. This is one of the reasons why conventional treatment (chemo and radiation) fails in 40 to 50 percent of cancer cases. It is also the critical reason for using coffee enemas. Coffee enemas are important and necessary in eliminating cancer, no matter what method is used.

For people who are serious about preventing or curing cancer, Otto Warburg proved that you need to stop all fermentation in your body cells.

That brings us to some very important steps:

1. Increase oxygen supply with ionic electromagnetic nutrients, supplements, exercise, and most of all, enzymes.

2. Increase intestinal absorption.

3. Increase raw, ionic, electromagnetic vegetable and fruit juices. (3 to 5 glasses/day).

4. Increase oxygen metabolizing supplements like L-arginine, turmeric, periwinkle, Ginkgo biloba, etc.

5. Take copious amounts of pancreatic enzymes like Wobenzym-N or Solozyme. Dr. Kelley took 15 to 18 tablets daily for his pancreatic cancer.

6. Eliminate bad bacteria, candida fungus, and other parasites, and increase the good intestinal bacteria in your gut.

To further prevent or cure cancer, you will also need to:

1. Clear away intestinal crusts (barriers) with okra, pepsin E-3, and coffee enemas.

2. Eliminate all sugars, red meat, carbohydrates, refined and processed foods.

3. Unravel sticky (homocysteine) blood (Johanna Budwig's formula).

4. Eliminate candida fungus, bad bacteria and parasites. 80 percent of all cancer is intertwined with candida.

5. Raise the acetic pH. Remember that cancer cells love sugar (used for fermentation) and red meat, both very acetic.

6. Chronic acetic bodies (low pH) create changes in the cell mitochondria.

7. Oxygen is the "nuclear energy" of the body.

Dr. Johanna Budwig followed up on Dr. Warburg's findings. She continued working on Dr. Warburg's discovery about low acidity, glucose fermentation, elimination of all sugars, and low oxygen in cancer cells. She discovered that low, cationic pH (high acidity) and low oxygen in the blood, body cells, and cancer cells could be eliminated, and many people could become cancer-free. Her raw, fresh diet routine and vegetable juices, together with suppression of sugar, sugar substitutes, and preservatives, releasing sticky red blood cells, sunshine, and high vitamin C cures more than 85 percent of cancer patients.

From her microscope work she saw that almost all of the cancer patients had homocysteine-saturated sticky blood. The red blood cells were stuck together in rouleaux instead of separate. She discovered that using a mixture of flaxseeds crushed in a coffee grinder, flaxseed oil (polyunsaturated oils), plus quark and cottage cheese would unwind the blood and enable the blood cells to separate, giving them the ability to carry oxygen to the cancer and body cells.

This procedure was also combined with high-pH, anionic (alkaline) foods, fermented foods, pancreatic enzymes, fresh raw vegetables, fruits, raw nuts, and coffee enemas, plus restriction of all processed, sugar, carbohydrates and cationic foods. After treating over 2,500 patients, she acquired an 85 percent cure rate, with patients living more than 5 years.

Although Dr. Budwig died in 2000, her clinic in Germany is still treating cancer patients with the Budwig protocol. Many other alternative cancer-treating physicians in Germany also use her protocol. We suggest that if you use any alternative cancer cure methods, you consult with your cancer physician or oncologist, but also check on your computer about Dr. Budwig, an alternative cancer practitioner. It is wise to remember that these procedures can be used when people have regular chemotherapy, radiation and surgery treatment for the cancer cells.

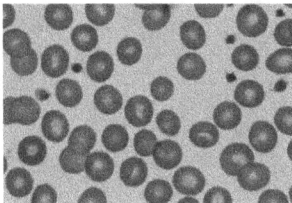

Free Blood

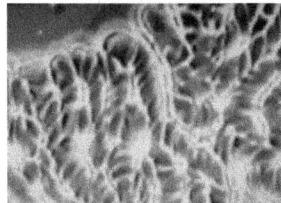

Sticky Blood

6

The Molecular World of Dr. Linus Pauling

There are not enough accolades that can be said about Dr. Linus Pauling.4a He was one of the most influential and knowledgeable scientists of all time Pauling's work, because of his chemical, mathematical and physics background has touched almost every chemistry student, medical doctor, and ordinary person since his discoveries on nutrition, chemical bonds, vitamin C, genetic diseases, physical structures of molecules, the double helix in molecular bonding and much more. He made important discoveries in so many fields that it leaves a person speechless.

In chemistry, physics, biochemistry, theoretical and applied medicine, Dr. Pauling made some very important discoveries in physical structures of molecular substances, nutritional therapy, chemical bonding, genetic diseases, vitamin C chemotherapy, cancer treatment, molecular evolution, and many other fields. His knowledge and dedication plus his work ethic led him into a physical and mathematical realm where he understood molecular structure, chemical properties, anion/cation relationships, and innovative principles relating to bond networks, structural geometry, DNA, RNA, the resonance of molecules and much more.

Pauling's discoveries and concepts led him to produce a book, still used by many chemistry students and physicians. In 1939 he published, "The Nature of the Chemical Bond, and the Structure of Molecules and Crystals." It was a classic and is still used today.

In 1948 working on a sudden insight and a sheet of paper, he discovered that a polypeptide chain, formed from amino acids, would coil into a helix structure he called "the alpha helix." The alpha helix is both a globular and fibrous protein that contributes nutritionally to many advances in nutrition and healing. Although he did not get credit for this discovery, he discovered the formula before two other men who got the Nobel prize for this achievement. He was held up in traveling to England to put in his discovery. Dr. Joanna Budwig later used his information to create a food combination to unravel "sticky" blood in the treatment of cancer.

In 1954 Dr. Pauling won the Nobel prize for his work on chemical bonding and modern structural chemistry. His scientific writings involved more than 350 publications, while his many discoveries help people all over the world lead better, healthier, longer, and more reproductive lives.

His work on Vitamin C was a revelation. The FDA and the drug companies called him a quack at the time. But now we know that he had discovered something revolutionary. It is a fact that in high doses, intravenous vitamin C produces hydrogen hydroxide, which is toxic to cancer cells.

The FDA and drug companies tried to dupe the public about Dr. Pauling's discoveries. Today it is coming out and you can find out more at; www.aacam.org. If you now have cancer, you might talk to your oncologist about adding IV vitamin C to your chemo cancer treatment. The following exciting story will show the positive effects of vitamin C. Several physicians and biochemists have now proven the treatment to be very effective

.

7

Dr. Linus Pauling and His Huge Discoveries About Vitamin C

Linus Pauling got two Nobel prizes. One was for his work in medicine, and the other was the Nobel peace prize. Neither was because of his great discoveries about vitamin C. It was not until 1984, ten years after his death, that new studies demonstrated that vitamin C was very helpful for human health, and that it was helpful in treating cancer and heart disease.

Most animals produce vitamin C. However, humans are not able to do so. They have to get vitamin C from the foods they eat and drink. The medical establishment fought tooth and nail to blunt the effect of Dr. Pauling's claims about vitamin C. His discovery was that intravenous vitamin C, in doses larger than 2,000 milligrams, helped slow or eradicate many diseases, including cancer, heart disease, and infections. He explained his research and findings in a book called Vitamin C and the Common Cold (1976).

The medical establishment tried to refute Pauling's claims. They conducted many trials where they tried to disprove his claim that high dosages of vitamin C would destroy cancer cells and treat heart disease. However, their research was flawed.

This is the same scenario that the medical establishment is using to discourage and fight the alternative treatment of cancer. The medical establishment and drug companies are still saying alternative treatments for cancer do not work and that doctors who use them are quacks.

The medical establishment tried to disprove Dr. Pauling's work about vitamin C. They said it was flawed and bogus. This was not new, as the medical establishment does not like anyone trying to change their drug, chemo, surgery and radiation treatment. Recent investigations by Drs. Steve Hickey and Hilary Roberts have shown some interesting findings that refute the medical establishment's previous investigation.

They found that the medical establishment's vitamin C studies and the National Institute of Health's studies were incorrect. In trying to refute Dr. Pauling's work, these institutions had used incorrect procedures and flawed data. The investigative work of Drs. Hickey and Roberts is published in a book called Ascorbate: the Science of Vitamin C (Hickey 2004). The book has 575 references. There probably is not any vitamin with so many incredible and effective uses in the world. This master nutrient helps ward off and cure, not one, but scores of diseases. Vitamin C even crosses the blood-brain barrier to help protect brain cells. It will not cure but helps prevent dementia, and it helps stop and reverse depression, degeneration, and Alzheimer's disease.

There is a great deal more to the vitamin C story. Its uses are astounding. It can even add years to a person's life.

Here are some of the treatments and diseases that this magic nutrient can help.

1 It is the best cold medicine on the planet.

2. It can help treat many chronic diseases such as diabetes, heart disease, and Alzheimer's disease. A 2019 study found vitamin C reduced high blood pressure (HBP) in diabetes patients. (reference?) In most diabetes patients it cut HBP in half.

3. It can defeat almost any infection.

4. For cancer, using IV therapy, it helps cure most cancers.

5. If cancer patients do not use IV therapy, they can help conventional treatment by taking 6,000 mg a day. Once inside cancer cells, vitamin C helps produce hydrogen peroxide, which is death to cancer cells.

6. It is an adjunct to help treat all chronic diseases.

7. Vitamin C reduces a person's cholesterol and LDL.

8. It keeps your telomeres shorter (See chapter 15).

These are many of the reasons why you should be taking 2,000 to 6,000 mg of vitamin C each day.

8

Dr. Carey Reams and the Reams Biological Theory of Ionization (RBTI)

The Reams Biological Theory of Ionization (RBTI) is a very important comprehensive test of factors that provide an understanding of the electromagnetic and biological systems in the human body. Very few people understand the important electromagnetic processes at work within the human body. The RBTI test provides the information necessary to address the cause of electrochemical and electromagnetic dysfunctions and sets up a program to reverse them. It is the missing link in diagnosing disease. Most people do not realize how important it is, and very few study and use this important test.

To use the Reams Biological Theory of Ionization test, fresh samples of urine and saliva are needed. The urine and saliva samples provide seven individual tests. They analyze the pH, conductivity of the body, cell debris, nitrate-nitrogen, and ammonia in the urine and the saliva.

The results of these tests, when analyzed, not only reveal the foundational cause of degenerative disease, but also reveal how to construct a diet and lifestyle to help find the electrochemical cause, and prevent these diseases before they occur.

Dr. Reams 5a had discovered that all biological entities (cells), whether plant, animal, or human, exist and function on their own basic unique electrochemical and electromagnetic frequency. He found that if the ionic mineral energy, moving into or out of a biological entity (body), is not in the proper frequency and conformity, that biological entity cannot maintain its ideal molecular, ionic, electrochemical, and electromagnetic structural integrity. Therefore, its health and physical well-being will degenerate accordingly. Dr. Reams discovered that the nutrient mineral density of our foods directly affects the quality of a human's or animal's digestive capability and that digestive integrity is required to maintain the ideal electrochemical and electromagnetic body frequency to maintain health and prevent degenerative disease.

To get accurate urine and saliva pH tests, a person should perform the Reams test one and one-half hours after breakfast, or one hour after lunch. That is when the liver is functioning under a meal when it is at its greatest potential.

Dr. Ream's approach: Dr. Reams openly insisted that the RBTI test was not a system of diagnosis. It is used for analyzing and determining what aspects of body chemistry need to be changed through a person's diet and lifestyle. It points the way to the things a person needs to eat, drink, breathe, think, and do to restore ideal health.

The energy within food is dependent on how much mineral and electromagnetic energy it contains. Testing hundreds of foods, Dr. Reams found that all foods are cationic except lemons. When foods enter the digestive tract, the anionic enzymes change the electrochemical, (pH) balance, which then activates electromagnetic foods to be able to supply the ionic cells and create energy. Most foods that are non-electromagnetic remain cationic and produce no energy. If in abundance, they also produce acidic cells, toxins, inflammation in the intestines, and disease.

The RBTI test is used to treat illnesses before they occur, and even before they show symptoms. The prime purpose of analyzing the biochemistry of the body is to create a diet and lifestyle program to promote perfect health. It was never used to diagnose or treat a disease. Only licensed medical practitioners are allowed to diagnose or treat disease. If a health practitioner is never exposed to the significance of Reams's RBTI principles, they will always and only have a symptom-based therapy system, no matter how natural their orientation. Many times, they will also miss finding the original cause.

Dr. Jim Daily, a biochemist and supplement manufacturer (Daily Manufacturing), produces many of the Reams dietary supplements.

Preventing disease is not about keeping the pH of your body alkaline. The alkalinity of the body does not assure the prevention of any disease or guarantee any person's health. Many disease conditions are related to an alkaline body. The RBTI test is for the primary purpose of analyzing and determining what is needed in a person's diet and lifestyle to maintain perfect health. That information can then be used to change the diet, to produce a more optimum pH range of 6.4.

9

How Important Are Vitamins, Minerals, and Supplements?

Researchers and many physicians have concluded that most adults over 50 do not consume an optimal amount of vitamins, minerals, and supplements from food sources alone.

As a person gets older, their body does not metabolize foods as well as a younger person's. Vitamins, minerals, and other nutrients are the insurance one needs to stay healthy. They include the antioxidants needed to help combat free-radical cell and organ damage and help stop inflammation. They can help to provide oxygen. They also minimize the effects of aging.

Well known U.S. physicians, such as Russell Blaylock, David Brownfield, Chauncey Crowell, and others, state that three out of five adults over 50 do not get enough vitamins and minerals.

Some of the more important supplements are magnesium, calcium, zinc, vitamin D3, B vitamins, vitamin C, chromium, niacin, iodine, vitamin E, B6, B12, CoQ10, turmeric, L-arginine, Ginkgo biloba, and folate.

Many well-known drug companies make inexpensive vitamins, minerals, and other supplements. Companies such as Pfizer, Bayer, GlaxoSmithKline, Novartis, and Unilever are a few of the big supplement manufacturers. The supplements that some companies make may be questionable, as the FDA often turns a blind eye, and does not require quality and label control or restrictions. The FDA rules, covering manufacturing quality, usually do not apply to vitamins, minerals, and most supplements.

I recommend two companies that are highly regarded for the quality, honesty, and integrity of their products. They are Daily Manufacturing and Standard Process. Daily Manufacturing is a company that a biochemist, Jim Daily, started, and produces the products that Dr. Carey Reams recommended, as well as many other great quality products. Jim Daily also lectures about supplements and body biochemistry. More information can be found on his website. Their address is 4820 Pless Road, Rockwell, NC 28138. Their phone number is (800) 782 7326. Check with your naturopath for Standard Process products, or check for their representatives online.

10

Food Vibrations

Many nutritionists and naturopaths rate foods by the vibrations they produce. Food vibrations are based on the fact that all matter contains vibration waves from light energy. These waves can be electrically measured. All live plants and animals produce vibration waves that are in turn produced in the plants and trees by the sun. This is especially true of foods grown outdoors in the soil, as vibrations are created by light waves.

All foods, then, can be tested with an electrical unit, and yield vibratory measurements from zero to thirty Hertz (Hz). Most refined and processed foods, canned foods, sugar products, and GMO foods register zero Hz, while raw soil-grown foods are rated much higher, from 27 to 30 Hz. We can connect the electromagnetic properties of ionic foods to their vibrations because both the ionic properties of foods and vibration have to do with electromagnetic energy.

Cationic, non-electromagnetic foods also measure at low or zero Hertz, because they have little or no energy, the same as other low-frequency-vibration food. Along with non-electromagnetic foods, sometimes no-vibration or zero-Hertz foods have been referred to as "dead" foods because they produce no energy.

The highest-vibration foods are raw fresh fruits, vegetables, nuts, sprouts, berries, leaves, bulbs, and other foods grown in the soil. The high vibration energy and frequency of these foods resonate with our blood, organs, and body cells, creating an energy force that will increase the disease-fighting ability of our immune system, intestinal bacteria, blood, organs, and body cells. The low-vibration foods, on the other hand, produce lower energy or no energy and will cause problems with our health and well being.

Organic fresh vegetables, fruits, berries, sprouts, and nuts can register the highest frequency vibrations, from twenty-five to thirty Hertz, while processed foods, refined foods, canned foods, vegetable oils, and GMO products have very little or no vibrations. Most of the latter are non-electromagnetic, cationic foods. For additional information on food vibrations and frequencies, there is a very informational book written by Robin Openshaw. It is called "VIBE," and tells about unlocking the energy frequencies of food, providing limitless health, love, and success.

11

Why You Should Consider Fermented Foods in Your Diet

The trillions of good bacteria in your small intestine are the hosts of good nutrition and health. You must be good to these bacteria, because not only do they comprise 80 percent of your immune system, they control your health and/or disease, from the food you eat.

If you want to stay healthy and free of disease, fermented foods should be on your daily food intake list. They help produce high ionic energy for your whole body and great food for the mighty immune bacterial giants in your small intestine. These mighty probiotic foods are the assisting foundation for your bacteria, immunity, health, and longevity. This is why fermented foods should be considered to be high on your everyday food list.

Fermenting has been one of the oldest forms of preserving food, dating back to more than 8,000 years. Many people from different countries depended on fermented food before refrigeration was even invented.

Most fermented foods are enriched with proteins, amino acids, vitamins, and also fatty acids. They are not only great probiotics but raise the pH and help stabilize the saliva, urine, and body cells.

High consumption of fermented foods is not recommended, but one to two small servings a day (especially before bedtime), could help raise an acid pH, plus could be a great benefit to your health and immune system. Kimchi, sauerkraut, plain yogurt, kefir, miso, kombucha, cottage cheese, and many other fermented foods greatly enhance your digestion, help chase out bad bacteria from your small intestine, plus are a great help to keep your acid/alkaline pH balance. Some great benefits of these probiotics are mentioned below:

1. Sauerkraut; sauerkraut is one of the oldest and most recognized fermented food. Captain Cook used it to prevent scurvy for his sailors when they traveled the high seas. Have you ever thought of eating it cold? One teaspoon or tablespoon a day is not only a probiotic enhancer but an alkaline helper for acidic bodies. It also is a stimulant for other "good bugs' and helps them multiply

2. Plain yogurt; plain yogurt is one of the best probiotics, but beware of flavored and colored brands. The best yogurt available is one filled with "live and active" cultures of bacteria. Please make sure that your yogurt is labeled to show "plain" and, if possible "live and cultured' bacteria. That kind can be gotten most of the time at the health food stores. Live and cultured yogurts usually have more than 100 million tiny good creatures that help chase out the bad bacteria in your gut.

3. Kimchi: Kimchi is another great fermented food. It creates great families of good bacteria (probiotics) while raising the alkaline balance in your body. Just one to two tablespoons before bedtime of cold kimchi will help increase your immunity while helping many happy good creatures multiple and help maintain a neutral pH.

4. Quark: I have mentioned quark many times in my book. It is great fermented food, helps create great numbers of good bacteria, and also does a miracle in your blood. Mixed with cottage cheese and flaxseeds (crushed) and/or flaxseed oil, it separates sticky (homocysteine) blood and increases the oxygen supply, while lowering the blood pressure. It also separates the blood cells, helping to increase oxygen, prevent clots (heart attacks, strokes, and clots in the veins). The author uses this formula for breakfast every day of the week to prevent cancer and heart disease. If you are interested in helping treat cancer and/or prevention of disease, this may be a serious consideration.

5. Cottage cheese; I don't need to give any more praising about cottage cheese. It not only helps produce millions of

good bacteria but is great alkaline food. As mentioned above with quark, crushed flaxseeds, and flaxseed oil works miracles for your health. Joanna Budwig's recommend recipe (chapter 26) is worth taking 4 to 5 times a week. especially for your blood, oxygen, and cell health.

6. Other great fermented probiotic, alkaline foods: miso, tempeh, appam, kombucha, fermented milk products that are fermented with lactic acid bacteria, such as lactobacillus and bacterium, champagne, Limburger cheese, sourdough bread, and others.

You can also easily make cultured, fermented foods. It is a great way to use up vegetables in your refrigerator with sea salt and vinegar. Your computer will get you on the path to making some great, healthy fermented probiotics.

12

Five Foods You Should Have Every Day

There are five important foods that are so important to your diet that it would be wise to try and have them every day. More information about these five foods will be discussed in section two of the book.

The Lemon

Almost all nutritionists, naturopaths, and physicians say that lemons and lemon juice are a great, great food. The evidence is overwhelming, since it is involved in more than 300 enzymatic reactions, and provides lots of vitamin C (ascorbic acid). The good things it does are amazing.

Although the lemon is very acidic, it will initiate the creation of alkaline enzymes in the body. This is extremely important since most people's saliva, urine, and body cells are acidic (cationic) and in the negative pH range. Dr. Carey Reams stated that two to three tablespoons of fresh-squeezed lemons with 1 cup distilled water every night before bedtime, plus every morning will help to bring the body pH higher, and in a better pH range. Even if your body is already at a normal pH, lemon juice will not usually make your alkalinity higher.

An acidic body is a platform where inflammation and radical cell damage can occur. Keeping the pH in the normal range helps reduce inflammation, radical cell damage, candida invasion, and disease. Also, it helps keep a healthier strain of bacteria in the intestines. Vitamin C does many other good things for your health.

Some of these other great things are:

1. It was found to prevent scurvy in sailors in ships starting many, many years ago. Capt. Cook was one of the first to give the sailors sauerkraut (vitamin C) to prevent scurvy. Sauerkraut is also a great probiotic.

2. Dr. Linus Pauling wrote in his book about vitamin C. He stated that vitamin C helped people get rid of colds and even showed that intravenous vitamin C helped to cure cancer and other diseases.

3. It helps prevent cancer.

4. Helps in the prevention of chronic diseases.

5. It enhances iron absorption.

6. Helps control blood pressure.

7. Neutralizes stomach acid and improves digestion

8. Helps the immune system in several ways. These benefits and more are reasons that I suggest using lemon juice twice a day and 2000 - 3000 mg. of vitamin C every day.

Garlic

Raw garlic should be the number 1 food we consume every day. But you say: "Isn't it bitter and makes your breath smell?" Yes and no! It isn't bitter if it is crushed or squeezed and put in your food, especially if you have enough food to dilute the garlic.

Chopping, crushing, and squeezing in a garlic squeezer releases the "allicin." which does miracle reactions in your body. Also, no one was ever hurt by a person's breath. Some books say garlic breath attracts women!

Cooking garlic reduces allicin's effectiveness, although it still has some good properties. I prefer 4-5 squeezed raw garlic cloves every day, as it is one of the greatest healthful foods.

Some of the wonderful benefits of garlic are:

1 .It is a good anticoagulant.

2. Boosts your digestion.

3. Helps neutralize stomach acid.

4 .Improves the oxygen intake to your cells.

5. Helps your circulation.

6. Is a great help to your immune system.

7. Helps control Candida albicans fungus and parasites.

8. It kills bad bacteria. It was used as an antibiotic before antibiotics were introduced.

9. Helps produce important digestive enzymes.

10. Increases brain function.

11. Besides killing many species of bad bacteria, it kills many species of viruses and candida.

12. Helps produce NO_2 (nitric oxide), which helps blood pressure.

My suggestion: Take four to five squeezed or chopped cloves of garlic every day, crushed and mixed with your food.

Turmeric

Recently, researchers have found some incredible reasons for everyone to take turmeric every day. First, turmeric has a unique ingredient called "curcumin" (also in curry). It is a powerful compound that combats inflammation and free radical reactions in the body cells. The unique ability to fight inflammation and free radical cell damage is just the start of many incredible benefits. Toxins, inflammation, and radical cell damage are the root cause of almost every human disease.

Turmeric (curcumin, curry) also helps the body in these other ways.

1. Helps high blood pressure, heart disease.

2. Helps prevent dementia and help a person think more clearly.

3. Helps slow and prevent arthritis.

4. Helps with memory retention.

5. Helps reduce cholesterol.

6. Promotes healthy digestion.

7. Reduces homocysteine (blood clotting factor), and has many more benefits.

A person can make turmeric and cinnamon tablets. Buy turmeric powder (and cinnamon powder if desired) from the health food store. Buy a jar of 500 No. 2 empty capsules from the drug store. Purchase a 50-unit capsule maker from an online retailer like Amazon, and you are in business. This saves way more than buying turmeric tablets for about $1.00 each. I suggest each person take two to three tablets a day.

Cold Raw Polyunsaturated Oil

Perhaps you have heard, "An apple a day keeps the doctor away." Well, raw polyunsaturated oils could use the same slogan. "A tablespoon a day will keep heart attacks away." That is how important this oil is.

What are cold polyunsaturated oils, and why are they so important? It is because of the makeup of the molecule. "Poly" means double or more. This means that these oils are made up of double helix bond molecules, They are essential for stopping inflammation, free free-radical cell damage, unhealthy blood, disease, and poor health. Most polyunsaturated oils come from raw (remember, raw!) northern seed oils, flax, borage, fish, marine species, eggs, and other seeds. These omega-3 oils are divided into three types. All are very beneficial in the prevention of disease: eicosapentaenoic acid (EPA), which is found in fish and ocean species, alpha-linolenic acid (ALA), extracted from raw northern seed oils, nuts, olives, flaxseeds, pumpkin, hemp, and grape seeds, plus a third oil, docosahexaenoic acid (DHA), also found in fish and marine species, as well as in the yolks of eggs.

These oils are more healthful when not heated. Cooking, heating or boiling an oil can slowly change it from an omega-3 oil to an omega-6 oil. That is why all oils on the grocery shelf are not anionic but cationic (boiled dead oils). One exception is extra virgin olive oil, but it shouldn't stay on the grocery shelf long, and must be in a dark bottle to stay as a polyunsaturated (omega-3) oil. All omega-3 oils need to be kept cold to maintain the double bond molecules. The reason is that when warmed, heated or cooked, they lose some or all of their anionic, healthy, body-metabolic function ability.

Essential raw oils support a number of wonderful body functions. A very important mission is to dissolve vitamins for use in the body. Omega-6 (dead) vegetable oils will not do that. In fact, they are completely cationic, and when used in excess, are an important cause of much severe inflammatory and free-radical cell damage, which contributes to arthritis, high blood pressure, heart disease, and even cancer.

Another very important function of polyunsaturated oils is that they improve blood circulation and oxygen flow. Recent research has found that using flaxseed oil with chemotherapy significantly enhances the effectiveness of chemotherapy in killing cancer cells. This is very important in cancer treatment. As mentioned before, cancer loves a low- to no-oxygen environment.

Recently, News Max and Dr. Russell Blaylock, in a book entitled " Cancer Survival Guide," wrote about Johanna Budwig's crushed flaxseeds, flaxseed oil, quark (fermented goat's milk), and cottage cheese mixture, used to unravel sticky (rouleau) blood and allow more oxygen to flow through the body. This helps immensely in reducing and eliminating cancer cells. Also, for one to prevent cancer, it is a good policy to use this flaxseed/quark/cottage cheese mixture to create better oxygen utilization, keep blood unraveled, and help lower blood pressure, (Rx: four to seven times a week).

I suggest 1 tablespoon of flaxseeds (crushed in a coffee grinder) plus 2 tablespoons flaxseed oil, fish oil or other polyunsaturated oil, mixed with quark, cottage cheese and crushed garlic. Mix in a few cut-up fruits or berries for taste. Restrain from using vegetable (dead) oils from the grocery shelf.

7-11 Fresh Fruits and Vegetables Every Day

The use of non electromagnetic (dead) foods for breakfast almost every day is practiced in fifty to sixty percent of U.S. households. Non-electromagnetic breakfast cereals and pasteurized milk are commonplace. Cationic sugared breakfast cereal and refined fast food products are going off the grocery shelves like rain in a cloudburst. Fast food and processed and refined foods make up the majority of the diet for many families. Bread, potatoes, and starchy foods are daily present on many dinner tables. This is one of the reasons that the cost of medical treatment in the US is far above almost every country in the world. The ratio of US medical cost is ten times higher per person than in China. Cancer in the US is rampant. The regimen of non-electromagnetic foods that make up an acidic diet is the mainstay for the majority of families in our North American world.

It is no wonder that seven to eleven fresh fruits and vegetables may seem a bit much, but believe me, the vegetables and fruits should be the focal point and the electromagnetic, ionic energy boost of your day. They pack so much energy, it is amazing. Veggies and fruits produce many vitamins, enzymes, minerals, amino acids, fiber, and other nutrients. They create great intestinal bacteria. Biochemists no longer think that five fruits and veggies give enough of these important electromagnetic anions to combat cancer, diabetes, HBP and other forms of disease. If you think of it, for breakfast it is easy to put four to five raw, fresh, cut-up fruits, berries, and melons in your bowl. As I do, you might add a few raw walnuts, almonds, and pecans. Then, if you want to get brave, add some cottage cheese, quark, flaxseeds. or flaxseed oil. That will jump-start your day, three to seven times a week. In the evening, raw veggies or a salad with six to seven veggies is not too much. A person can add chopped or boiled eggs, veggies, beans, or wild-caught fish. Eggs are healthful for breakfast. You may think of lightly boiled eggs, plus added nuts, chopped veggies, and even garlic, if you want to stay healthy.

This is a wonderful story, about the longest-living person who died in 2017. She was 117 years old. For more than 50 years, until she died, she ate two raw eggs for breakfast every day. She knew that eggs must be good for you.

Besides the eggs, you can alter your breakfast with rye or oatmeal mush, sprinkled with fresh fruits, grapes, berries, bananas, raisins, dried cranberries, etc. Beans, fish, and chicken can be the protein that a healthy family eats, three to four times a week.

Your breakfast should be the most important energy-producing meal of the day. Breakfast cereals, processed and refined foods just don't hack it. If you want to stay healthy, think "live ionic food, not dead cationic food." You can strengthen your immunity when you follow up breakfast with an electromagnetic, live-food diet the rest of the day. With this diet, your trips to the doctor will be like eating an apple a day. In a perfect world, you will be far ahead of the masses.

13

Your Immune System: Could 80 Percent of all Cancers be Related to Candida?

ASSOCIATES (intestinal bacteria or microbiome) can be tiny workers that work for compensation. What is their compensation? Health and longevity for both you and your friendly 25 plus trillion intestinal bacteria. Next point: You may not think about it, but you have two and one half to four lbs. of hard-working, small intestinal guests (ASSOCIATES) that you feed every day. Are you feeding them healthy nutritious raw food with pure water, vitamins, minerals, enzymes, amino acids, and polyunsaturated oils? All of these nutrients are needed for your trillions of health workers to keep you and them healthy and free of disease.

Did you know that scientists have discovered that candida fungus in your intestines is associated with 80 percent of cancers? This is a terrifying statement about your intestinal bacteria and association with candida fungus. Incredible new research suggests that a common, little known fungus could be an important factor in the formation of the cancer process. A recent research article, "Critical Reviews in Microbiology," states that candida Albicans fungus is capable of promoting cancers by several mechanisms. This is very important research, as most oncologists never even mention candida and the serious result of having an infestation in your small intestine. Dr. Milton White states that as many as 220 million people in the U.S. may have an overgrowth of candida fungus in their small intestines. This means that candidiasis is probably the most important enemy of your body, intestinal flora, and the immune system. Symptoms of candida and candidiasis are thrush, nail fungus, jock itch, vaginitis, crust on nails, and/or heels. Most people do not show any symptoms. Your diet determines the amount of candida in your intestines. That is why a good diet is so important.

Do you know about symbiosis? It is the relationship between you and your intestinal bacteria. Helping each other is a symbiotic relationship.

However, when the host (you) eats a lot of non-electromagnetic, non-electrochemical, refined, and processed acidic foods, the symbiosis gets distorted and the intestinal bacteria get weak, some die, and others cannot do their function of helping to digest food and keep bad enemies away. You, too, are involved, because you have no intestinal insurance and lose your intestinal workers protection. Once lost, you also get exposed to candida fungus, parasites, toxins, intestinal inflammation, leaky gut, radical blood, body cell, and organ changes which cause autoimmune and other diseases. They creep through your armor and create havoc. The importance of your intestinal bacteria cannot be underestimated.

We might say, "If you want to help me, I must help you." It's a 50-50 man/bacteria symbiosis.

The bacteria in your immune system are responsible to help digest your food and combat bad bacteria, viruses, and parasites that are trying to destroy your health and longevity. But what other bacteria, parasites, cells, and organs are involved? Why is your diet so critical for these little health workers? What happens when you are eating a chronic bad non-electromagnetic acidic diet? These are all very important questions that people should know and understand.

Between 2008 and 2012, the Human Microbiome Project studied the microscopic organisms that live in our bodies. What they found is that a person's body of 25 plus trillion cells is the home of 800 different microbe strains. These microbes have an enormous effect on our health, immune system, mood, thinking, appetite, and even our appearance. They are like a virtual organ.

The action of these vital essential microbes is astonishing.

1. They act as our immune system, devouring bad germs.

2. They produce several vitamins, including vitamins K, B 12, thiamine, and riboflavin

3. They produce estrogen, melatonin, and estriol.

4. They break down food for energy.

5. They produce neurotransmitters, serotonin, dopamine, and norepinephrine.

6. They communicate with your heart and brain.

Bad intestinal bacteria, fungus, and parasites create most of the diseases in humans. The main cause is a dangerous condition of bad diet and over-acidity, which gives rise to an internal gut environment conducive and subject to bad bacteria, candidiasis, parasites, toxins, inflammation, cell wall breakdown, leaky gut, and disease. This bad diet plus acidic environment changes and weakens the 80 – 20 bacteria ratio, immune system, and/or the 25 plus trillion hard-working health workers. Toxins abound! With a bad diet, the good bacteria get weak, even into wars, and get destroyed by bad bacteria and parasites who try to outnumber them. That is when they lose their 80 percent - 20 percent ratio of good bacteria to bad bacteria. Bad bacteria, molds, viruses, and parasites including Candida Albicans, and other parasites weaken the good bacteria and their ability to fight and win the disease war for the host. Candida not only produce ethanol and many other toxins, poisons, and inflammation in the gut but attach themselves to normal healthy cells and wreck the DNA, which causes free radical cell damage, diseases, and even cancer.

To function properly, the immune system performs many duties. One of the most important duties is to detect and destroy a lot of bad guys (pathogens). These pathogens vary from bad bacteria to viruses, parasites, and even sometimes residual proteins and food particles that get into the blood system. They also fight the bad bacteria, parasites, and viruses in their own home (biome). The immune system does its magic by distinguishing between good and bad bacteria, viruses, and parasites. It attacks the enemy while keeping the family of good bacteria safe, healthy, and alive. However, these bacteria need to have a healthful supply line (you) bringing in new good nutrients, vitamins, enzymes, amino acids, minerals, and healthy (electromagnetic) oils.

Another great function of the immune system is to form immunity to certain diseases with what is called an antigen-antibody reaction. This is a process where the bacteria can recognize a disease like polio, smallpox, or mumps (often in vaccinations) and creates an antibody or continued immunity for that disease. This acquired immunity involves an immunological memory leading to a response from any red flag exposure to subsequent exposures from that same pathogen. A red flag exposure leads to an immediate maximal response by the immune system. It will act immediately, sometimes just by eating the bad culprits (phagocytosis). Other times it will create a body fever to assist in driving the pathogens out. The immune system can improve its recognition and elimination of the culprit with a high temperature.

To summarize, the primary role of the good bacteria and the immune system is:

1. Identify potential injurious and infectious bacteria, viruses, parasites, and other pathogens.

2. Assess the level of the threat and send out an army of white blood cells.

3. Mount a response to that threat, immobilize, neutralize or destroy the pathogens.

4. Repair any damage that occurs from the pathogens

5. Eat the food you give them to end up ionic and digest it while giving all the vitamins, minerals, amino acids, enzymes, oils, and other nutrients back to you through the villi in your small intestine, into your blood and body cells.

6. Good microbes from mother's milk are passed through to the baby. This is a great start for the baby to begin life with a great microbiome.

If your diet contains bad, non-electromagnetic, and dead food, it will cause an acidic or over alkalinity of the blood, body cells, and organs. In these conditions, these mighty little warriors will not be healthy enough to send good nutrients to the blood and body cells, so the toxins and waste materials get into your blood and create havoc with your body cells, heart, and brain. Then a person can get inflammation, leaky gut, radical cell damage, and disease. In many cases, pain is associated with the inflammatory process. This is especially true with arthritis and rheumatism patients.

The immune system bacteria need many nutrients, vitamins, enzymes, amino acids, good polyunsaturated and monounsaturated oils, minerals, and other supplements. One of the more important ones is vitamin C. Vitamin C is needed by all the white blood cells to maintain their protein controlling enzymes, which are needed to attack toxins plus bacteria and destroy them. Without Vitamin C, magnesium, and copper, white blood cells (leucocytes) will lose their macrophage (destroying) capabilities.

Other nutrients that help are calcium, vitamin D3, turmeric, cinnamon, lipoic acid, zinc, selenium, grape seed extract, omega 3 oils, and green tea. Calcium and magnesium activate blood cells.

High body temperature will increase the enzymatic augmentation of the immune and liver function. That is why many alternative cancer patients have a treatment that recommends hot baths. Stress suppresses the immune system.

One caution: Antibiotics destroy the good bacteria in your small intestine. This creates a barn door opening which not only leads to antibiotic-resistant bacteria but worse, with the barn door open, bad bacteria, candida, viruses, and other parasites sneak in, replacing the good bacteria. Subsequently, the candida and bad bacteria change the ratio of good bacteria (normal 80 percent) to bad bacteria (normal 20 percent), to maybe 70 to 30 percent, or worse yet, 60 to 40. This result is a weakening of the immune system, and the creation of a disease environment.

Auto-immune disease. Chronic gut toxins and inflammation in the small intestine are increasing in the United States. This is relative to the increase in obesity, fast-food diets, plus the increase in sugar, carbohydrates, red meat, vegetable oils, refined, processed, and non-electromagnetic acidic foods. The result of gut inflammation is a leaky gut. Leaky gut is responsible for Crone's disease, ulcerative colitis, and other diseases. Some of the results of these intestinal disease-producing conditions are asthma, rheumatoid arthritis, type 1 diabetes, atherosclerosis, multiple sclerosis, HBP, heart disease, brain disorders, and even cancer. One of the rising causes of auto-immune disease is a leaky gut and ulcerative colitis.

What is a leaky gut syndrome?

1. It is a weakening of the one–two cell walls of the small intestine, caused by toxins and inflammation in the small intestine.

2. Inflammation, infection, and breakdown of the cell wall create small holes in the lining leading into the blood.

3. Toxins, bad bacteria, candida, parasite larvae, protein molecules, and tiny food matter get into the blood. They send toxins to the body cells.

4. In the blood, they create a histamine reaction where white blood cells (leucocytes) proliferate and try to destroy the tyrants.

5. These toxins, bacteria, and protein particles produce leucocytosis, histamine, asthma, and many autoimmune diseases.

6. Histamine reactions, rash, itching of the eyes, low chronic fever, sinus drainage, headaches, and sinus infections may also occur.

7. Worse, toxins get into the blood. and go to the body cells. In large amounts, these toxins in body cells can change the mitochondria and cause many diseases, including heart disease, diabetes, cancer, and brain disease.

I mentioned previously that the bacteria in your small intestine create 80 percent of your white blood cells and immune activity. However, four other organs are involved and comprise the other 20 percent. They are the liver, thymus gland, bone marrow, and spleen. Leucocytes are formed in the spleen, while some other white blood cells are formed in the bone marrow.

Recent research has shown that the immune system can influence the brain. The intestinal bacteria can influence brain activities, behavior, and function. Some of these conditions are mood, depression, sugar cravings, food addiction, and restless sleep:

Small intestine toxins, inflammation, and leaky gut are the number one health destroyers in the U.S. It is estimated that 30 – 50 percent of all Americans have a leaky gut. A leaky gut can result in autoimmune diseases, inflammatory diseases, blood vessel plaque, diabetes, heart disease, obesity, and even cancer. It occurs when inflammatory toxins in the immune system flora are compromised with bad intestinal bacteria and Candida Albicans from a chronic acidic diet. Dr. David Brownstein 10a describes all this in his book: "Heal Your Leaky Gut."

Candida fungus infestation can go on for years. The candida infestation can show up in many seemingly healthy people that are suddenly diagnosed with auto-immune diseases, other diseases, and/ or cancer. Most people do not realize it, but with antibiotics, candida fungus can double in as little as 24 hours.

Substances that increase candida are:

Antibiotics

Vaccines

Surgery

Steroids

Chemotherapy

Drugs

Chronic non-electromagnetic acidic diet

Excess sugar

Excess (dead) vegetable oils, and 10. Excess red meat

Harvard researcher, Julia Koehler reports that "candida is, by far, the most predominant pathogen involved in human disease."

When you have symptoms such as thrush, toenail fungus, vaginitis, jock itch, or heavy crust on your heels, you may also have candida fungus in your small intestine. If you suspect you have candida fungus, get an antifungal from your physician, naturopath, or nutritionist and change your diet.

Antibiotics, including Cipro, with just one prescription, can devastate your good bacteria. Restoration may take as long as six months or a year. Maybe you should show this book to your dentist. Many do not realize the gut devastation that antibiotics cause.

14

The One Hundred Year Old Marathon Man

Recently, the newspapers ran a story about an interview with a hundred year-old man. What is so intriguing was that the man had just run a 26.2-mile marathon. When he was asked about the feat, he said that he still had a lot of energy, very acute vision, and thinking ability. There was no doubt that he also had a very strong and healthy body. He also stated that he ran more than 43, 500 miles in his lifetime, an incredible feat. When asked about his diet, the marathon man said: "I eat mostly fruits and vegetables, and stay away from desserts and sweet things."

This man was a great silent advertiser of exercise, oxygen, discipline, and an electromagnetic ionic diet. He is also silently saying that these things; exercise, vegetables, fruit, staying away from sugar, processed meats, dead vegetable oils, and discipline are probably the most important health advice anyone would ever receive. But if this is broken down into what might be the greatest factor in anyone's health, what would you think it might be? We need many things in our diet, but most physicians think it might be oxygen.

All vertebrates need oxygen to survive. Not getting enough oxygen through the day can be a significant drag on your health and longevity. The more of it, the better. Even many alternative cancer treatments now use hyperbaric oxygen and exercise as one of their many methods to cure cancer. Oxygen is a very important and vital thing for our health and very important for cancer patients.

Recent research has shown that the more oxygen a person gets, usually the healthier they are. Oxygen is important because it boosts the oxygen intake for the body cells. Body cells that are deprived of oxygen because of inflammation and free radical damage are subject to weakness, disease, and cancer. Increased oxygen helps keep the body cells healthy.

What researchers have found is that a poor diet and low cell oxygen leads to damage of your telomeres, which control how long your cells will last in your lifetime. A poor diet, intestinal inflammation, leaky gut, and free radical cell damage in the blood and body cells leads to changes in the DNA, RNA, mitochondria cell damage, disease, and telomere shortening.

These are several things that are related to energy, DNA damage, and telomeres:

- Stress

- Obesity

- Lack of exercise

- Lack of lung exercise

- Processed meats

- Sugar

- Dead oils

- Homocysteine in the blood (sticky blood and oxygen loss)

The 100 year-old marathon man might have been aware that these things were related to energy, shortening of a person's telomeres, and shortening of life.

An acetic, refined food, processed food, sugar, vegetable oil, and non-electromagnetic diet leads to radical changes in the blood vessels and red blood cells. It reduces their ability to carry oxygen. When this same diet routine continues, things get worse and worse. Lack of blood oxygen can damage the mitochondria in the body cells. The body cells do not get enough oxygen. The brain does not get enough oxygen. Plaque gets into the blood vessels. Sticky blood then continues to reduce the oxygen intake to the blood and body cells.

Putting this into perspective, all eight of the things mentioned above and more are vital to a person's health and longevity. Oxygen is very important, but must be combined with a good raw diet of fruit, vegetables, berries, leaves, melons, roots omega 3 oils, raw nuts, etc. plus staying away from sugar, carbohydrates, refined foods, processed meats, "dead" vegetable oils and prolonged sitting

These healthy foods also help in keeping your blood vessels open, reducing plaque and homocysteine (clotting factor). This allows the red blood cells to bring more oxygen to the body cells, organs, and just as important, to the intestinal bacteria, plus prolongs telomere shortening.

I have discussed the important findings of Dr. Joanna Budwig. She increased the oxygen intake to cancer patients by feeding them a mixture of quark, cottage cheese, flaxseed oil, and crushed flaxseeds. For prevention and cancer patients, taking this formula seven times a week can also be a great asset plus the added oxygen that a person's body cells get from exercise.

Another thing That needs to be considered is the air that you get in your workplace. So many businesses, while making their products, produce dust, chemicals, and/or toxins that can also reduce the oxygen intake to the body plus cause other health problems. If you work in one of these places, check to make sure proper safeguards are taken so you get a pure, good source of oxygen in the air.

Breathing exercises: Taking breathing exercises every day are also a very good way for a person to increase their oxygen intake. A good routine will be to pick a quiet time and take 5 big breaths. Not just ordinary breaths, but take in on each breath as much air as possible, then try to take in more. Hold for ten to twenty seconds, then release slowly. Then do this, three to four more times. If you do this routine a couple of times each day, it will help you increase your body oxygen.

There are also some great supplements you can take that are becoming very popular with the medical establishment. They are very high on my list of supplements. Researchers say that nitric oxide is very important for your body and helps to increase the oxygen supply. Nitric oxide helps relax and increase the size of your blood vessels, allowing more oxygen to flow through them. Four of these great supplements are L-arginine, Gingko Biloba, beetroot powder, L-citrulline, pycnogenol, garlic, and turmeric. That is why they are listed so high in my rating of supplements. I suggest you take some of these nitric oxide supplements every day.

I heartily compliment the extraordinary achievements of the marathon man. His telomeres were a little longer than normal due to his diet, exercise, and oxygen intake. He is living proof that diet, exercise, and oxygen are vital factors in disease prevention and longevity. I hope he will be an inspiration for every one of you reading this book. He is certainly one in a million, er, rather, one in 325 million.

15

Go Slow on Those Nasty Lectins

What are lectins? They are certain molecules in different foods that can initiate an irritation in your small intestine. Their origin is in some food plant cells that you consume. These lectins repel (resist) insects, bacteria, fungus, and molds in the plant foods as they are maturing. Some engineering firms even engineer certain plants to create lectins which will repel (resist) pests and certain herbicides.

The lectins are in many foods that you eat. They are in legumes, grains, soybeans, other beans, peanuts, grains, cashews, tomatoes, potatoes, and rice to name many of them.

Dr. Steven Gundry has recently brought the importance of lectins to the general public. He has written a book about lectins, called "The Plant Paradox." You may have also seen Dr. Gundry's videos on the computer and TV. His book states that lectins are a great danger to a person's health. The book even has the view that maybe we should not be eating lectins, or reduce them to a minimum.

Other Authors and researchers contest what Dr. Gunthry says about lectins being so dangerous. They state that his claims have not been backed by enough research to rule them out of your diet. Most lectins are not as dangerous as Dr. Gunthry states. Researchers have said that cooking lectins take out the biggest percentage of lectins from the vegetables, beans, and grains Most lectins are not as toxic to the gut wall as he states. In fact, by skipping lectins altogether, a person may end up with some nutritional deficiencies. It is only with excess or binge eating that lectins may be a problem. Some lectins may produce mild stress but can trigger a healing response. It is true that in humans, lectins, along with other toxins reduce the chemical protection along the intestinal wall that protects the thin gut lining. These chemicals are called cytokines. When cytokines are reduced, erosion of the gut wall (leaky gut) can occur. The resulting holes let inflammatory toxins, candida, protein particles, parasite larvae, and tiny food particles flow into the blood.

With so many foods having lectins, it is almost impossible to eliminate them. My purpose is to inform you of which foods are lectins and educate you so you will be able to make a rational decision about lectin toxicity. Also, it is important to know that raw lectin foods have many more lectins than cooked lectin foods.

Some beans and mushrooms contain anticancer phytochemicals. Many of these foods offering protection against cancer. What else besides the reduction of lectin foods helps decrease the toxicity of the gut wall?

Some of these things are:

1. Consume lots of polyphenols and vegetables.

2. Eat seven to eleven fresh foods, berries, and fruits every day.

3. Prevent nutritional and mineral deficiencies.

4. Keep your intestinal biome healthy and within the eighty to twenty percent good to bad bacteria ratio.

5. Eliminate sugar and sugar incorporated foods.

6. Try to be aware of eating less raw lectin foods including raw peanuts, cashews, soybeans, castor beans, raw kidney beans, potatoes, peanut butter, grains, and tomatos.

7. Eliminate all oils on the grocery shelf and cut down on all deep-fried foods.

8. Supplement with turmeric, L–arginine, and vitamin C, among others.

9. Keep your saliva and urine pH in the neutral zone, or slightly alkaline.

I hope this did not ruin your day. Lectins are still nutrient foods that help a person's metabolism, digestion, and immune system. Knowing about them is the first step. We might also remember that some of the oldest people on earth have been eating lectin foods for 90 years or more. They seem to be very healthy. I'm sure they haven't read Dr. Gunthry's book.

16

The Most Important and Unique Wall in the World

The most important and unique wall in the world is the one to the two-celled thin intestinal lining of your small intestine (gut wall). Not only is it responsible for keeping you healthy, but it determines the health of your body cells, organs, blood, heart, and even your brain. It also influences the health and protects your body, your ability to resist disease, also to think, adjust your heartbeat, and most of all your ability to live a long and prosperous life.

A reservoir of dendritic cells patrols the border of your gut wall. Chemicals called cytokines are released when toxins cause inflammation. They send macrophages (killer cells) to combat the toxins, protecting the intestinal cell wall. Excess toxins and inflammation will overwhelm the killer cells, and breach the thin intestinal wall, causing a leaky gut.

What makes the intestinal wall so important is that with a healthy diet, the cytokines, macrophages, and healthy bacteria (healthy microbiome) control the gut lining to keep it healthy. With a healthy gut wall, the healthy bacteria transfer oxygen, minerals, vitamins, enzymes, amino acids, and other nutrients through the thin cell wall and into the blood. In the blood, these nutrients do their magic and go to all the body cells and organs, keeping the body healthy and free of disease.

It all relates to the diet and the healthy microbes being vital and healthy. These 25+ trillion good, healthy bacteria are a person's greatest bosom friends. Keep good care of them.

When the diet is not good, and a person eats a chronic consumption of sugars, omega 6 vegetable oils, red meat, refined and processed foods, etc., things do not go so well. There is trouble in River City. The colonies of inflammatory toxins from the bad diet create holes in the very thin gut wall. They overwhelm the cytokines and macrophages. The dam breaks, opening the gate to bad terrorists (toxins, tiny food molecules, tiny protein molecules, bad bacteria, molds, and candida fungus). These holes, called leaky gut, even get bigger as the inflammatory toxins continue to erode the thin walls and deregulate the gut. This next part is scary. The toxins, endotoxins, bad bacteria, fungus, food and protein molecules, parasites, and polysaccharides escape into your blood and can travel in your blood to your heart, body cells, organs, and brain. This is the start of chronic disease states including autoimmune diseases plus serious ailments like HBP, heart disease, diabetes, cancer, dementia, and other brain disorders.

Microglial cells protect your brain from infections. The brain has a blood-brain barrier like the small intestinal lining. The lymph system takes out the waste. But here is the scary part. Microglial cells are the primary immune cells of the central nervous system. They act like cytokines and macrophages, responding to toxic pathogens and injury. An invasion of chemical toxins can overpower the microglial cells. When the microglial brain cells get overwhelmed, toxic bacteria and molecules then reach the blood-brain barrier and enter the brain. This is the start of dementia and brain disease.

Recent research has shown that although microglial and t-cells try to suppress inflammation in the brain, a swarm of inflammation toxins can pass through the blood-brain barrier and overwhelm the neurons, axons, and synapses. The synapse creates chemical connections involving acetylcholine to communicate and function. Chemical damage to the synapse occurs and is critical in altering brain function. It is now found that depression, dementia, Alzheimer's disease, Parkinson's disease, multiple sclerosis, sleep deprivation, and some other brain functions are all related to this debilitating toxic chemical disease process.

It all starts with the intestinal wall lining. That is why it is so important to have a good diet. It can be said that 90 percent of all diseases start with a bad diet. The inflammatory toxins that breach the gut lining create havoc on the joints, body cells, organs, heart, and even the brain. A healthy diet keeps the thin small intestinal walls strong and toxin resistant. That is why the gut wall is the most important and unique in the world. It also shows that the health of the small intestinal wall determines the health of the body cells, organs, immune system, and brain. If more people knew this, there would be fewer autoimmune diseases, other diseases, and more healthy brains, plus a lot less depression, dementia, Alzheimer's disease, Parkinson's disease, multiple sclerosis, sleep deprivation, and other brain function issues.

17

The Sugar and Oil Coated Four Lane Road to Cancer

By now you know that every person needs to create energy by the friction between anion and cation atoms, molecules, and cells. You know that to stay healthy a person also has to consume more raw and natural anionic foods than cationic foods, keeping cationic foods to a minimum. To stay healthy, it is wise to keep the pH of saliva and urine at 6.2 to 6.8. This regime keeps the cells, blood, body organs and intestinal bacteria healthy and full of energy.

But what has gone wrong in America? The average person produces way more cationic foods than anionic foods. This creates toxins, cell inflammation, leaky gut, dirty blood, and free radical cell damage. This allows bad bacteria and candida fungus to weaken the immune system. These foods, sugar, excess carbohydrates, processed and refined foods, omega 6 vegetable oils, and excess red meat are the biggest drivers of unhealthy eating. Overeating of these foods may cause immense damage to the intestines, body cells, blood, and body organs, and even the brain. Also, very important, they change the ratio and chemistry of the good/bad bacteria in the intestines.

Very few physicians, dentists, therapists, and worse yet, superintendents and instructors in schools take an interest in a student's or a person's diet and health. Yet Dr. Carey Ream's book states that the diet and choice of food intake are far more important than treating a person after he or she has an infection or disease from a poor diet or very poor choice of food and liquid intake. Teaching food choice and proper anion/cation food consumption will help young people, students and adults live a future with healthier food choices, better health, less disease, fewer trips to the physician and dentist plus great longevity.

McDonald's is probably one of the most successful restaurant businesses in America. It is the king of the cationic diet, using cationic heated (dead) vegetable oils, refined carbohydrates, and sugar-filled soda drinks. It sells millions of French fries, hamburgers, plus millions of gallons of soda to people in America every year. These drinks are mostly sugar-filled or diet (worse than sugar) sodas. All these sugars and oils form "transfats" and "mega trans," help change the energy system from healthy to unhealthy, creating bad intestinal bacteria, a weak immune system, intestinal inflammation, leaky gut, free radical body cells, disease, and, even in many cases, cancer.

Here are some astounding statistics on food consumption (PER PERSON) for all people in America EACH YEAR:

1) 90 containers of French fried potatoes per year.

2) 400 ounces of omega 6 oils in salad dressings, deep-fried foods, mayonnaise, red meat fat, bacon, sausage, and other saturated vegetable oil-containing foods.

3) 300 ounces of deep-fried fish, potatoes, chicken, doughnuts, etc., not counting the (fried in vegetable oil) foods, prepared in millions of households.

4) 22 teaspoons of sugar and sugar products, corn syrup, and preservatives each day (95 – 120 pounds per year).

Imagine that you are racing four cars down a four-lane road. One car runs on French fries, the second lane car runs on omega 6 oils, the third in row three, on 300 ounces of deep-fried chicken, potatoes, and fish. The fourth lane car runs on 100 pounds of sugar and sugar products.

These cars are also fueled by smoking, overprescribing of antibiotics, chemicals (in food, farm products, hair, plastics, etc.), preservatives, genetically modified foods, the environment, damaging hormones, GMO products, air pollution, and many drug company's products. Think about how fast these hot rods can reach the end of the track (road).

Going farther down the road we can correlate this consumption of sugar, omega 6 oils, excess red meat, and chronic toxins to intestinal inflammation, leaky gut, free radical cell damage, and disease.

When the chronic cationic cell, blood, and organ imbalance continues, many detrimental things start to occur that can lead to cancer. These enemies of health {sugar, processed foods and meats, refined foods, and omega 6 vegetable (dead) oils}, plus other cationic products change the electromagnetic energy field, create toxins, bad intestinal bacteria plus increase Candida Albicans fungus overgrowth, and even parasites. Many people gain weight. Body toxins start to overload the intestines, liver, pancreas, immune system, and brain. The toxins from the bad bacteria, candida, and other parasites overload the liver, pancreas, and gall bladder. This overwhelms the very organs that help prevent cancer plus help to cure cancer. Changes ensue, such as gut inflammation, leaky gut, Crohn's disease, leucocytosis, other diseases, immune system overload, gall bladder overload, etc.

As the road gets faster and steeper, toxins from the intestines create individual body cell wall resistance. Oxygen, nutrients, and minerals have trouble getting into the body cells. Retained CO_2 and wastes weaken the cells. Toxins cause the blood to get sticky, producing excess homocysteine, creating oxygen deprivation in the blood and body cells. This oxygen deprivation makes it easier for cell mitochondria to change their chromosomes, creating a cancer cell. Cations also increase and overwhelm the energy fields, making it easy for the DNA and RNA in the mitochondria to change from normal, creating a cancer cell hit or changing a normal cell to a cancer cell.

The end of the road: All of these changes create a candida/cancer symbiosis, where some researchers show that cancer is related to the Candida Albicans fungus about 80 percent of the time. Hilda Clark, with her great book about candida, parasites, and cancer, predicted a candida/cancer symbiosis many years ago, but very few realized this until recent research has shown that eighty percent of all cancers are interlaced with Candida Albicans fungus.

Catherine Shanahan, M.D., a heart specialist in Canada, researched and studied 225 stroke and heart attack victims who were just admitted to her hospital, 24 hours or less, before. She discovered the 90% of these patients had consumed fried or deep-fried "dead" vegetable oils within 24 hours of being admitted to the hospital. These "dead" oils are vicious because they "spike" the omega 6 to omega 3 ratio from normal, 2 : 1 or 3 : 1 to 30 : 1, and even up to 50 : 1. This consumption of chronic high saturated fats, high sugar, transfats, and mega trans oil diet is very damaging to your blood, body cells, and organs. My suggestion is to minimize your intake of deep-fried and fried foods.

Maybe a person should think twice about saturated fats, high sugar, transfats, and mega trans. They are very damaging to your blood, body cells, and organs. This is why it is wise to minimize eating deep-fried foods, or when frying that twelve-ounce T bone steak, or frequently ordering wieners, sausage, doughnuts, sugary desserts, fries, and sodas. Hopefully, by understanding the prelude to cancer, you will understand how you, your family, and your family relations may be able to prevent it.

For those who wish to use a preventive cancer diet plus have an immune system enhanced diet, I suggest a supplement that contains many important amino acids, the precursors of many pancreatic enzymes. It is called wobenzym-N, Garden of Life. This supplement helps boost the immune system and is a help in preventing arthritis and cancer. It can be obtained on many online websites. There are some rare, mild side effects. You may get diarrhea and possible allergies, but overall, it is a great supplement. My wife and I take 3 tablets a day of wobenzym-N. We never have had any side effects.

I hope you can keep your unhealthy cars (unhealthy diet) off the road.

18

Oral Cavity: Incubator for Heart Disease and Cancer

Many people have not realized that 75 percent of all diseases are related to your mouth and oral health. Most diseases start and are critically related to tooth cavities and oral cavity infections. Experts are finding that infections in the mouth are a contributing and direct link in the transmission of heart disease and other diseases of the body. Oral infections, cavities, a person's uneven bite, root canals, metal poisoning, and a faulty temporal-mandibular joint all contribute to many body diseases, skeletal and muscular malfunctions.

Between 1,600,000 and 2,500,000, U.S. citizens die each year from heart disease and cancer. Another startling statistic is that only 6,000 die by being murdered by guns. Both of these statistics are very concerning. We cannot overlook both of them, but when you look a heart disease (735,000 deaths/year) and strokes (750,000 deaths/year), you can understand the problem that relates to oral health disease. An overwhelming amount of chronic daily toxins come from infections and bacteria in the oral cavity. The toxins are oxidative enemy agents, which produce a flood of new debilitating inflammation and radical oxidative cell damage.

These toxins come from infections, bad bacteria, candida fungus (thrush), viruses, infectious gums, tooth decay, tooth abscesses, tonsil abscesses, infected wisdom teeth, mercury, other metals, and root canals. Many of these ailments relate to toothaches, headaches, neck aches, pain, swelling, thrush, muscle aches, fatigue, mouth cancer, and much more.

The toxins from metals, bacteria, candida, and viruses produce a tremendous disease state in a neglected oral hygiene mouth because the temperature makes it an excellent bacterial growing laboratory.

Recently, many physicians, dentists, and researchers are saying that dental infections, infected teeth, infected gums, and injurious metals are the single reason for the flood of toxins that are the underlying cause of heart disease. This is a big statement, but recent research is showing that along with an acetic low body cell pH, the enormous oral health toxin overload creates several problems. This is why a person should keep their mouth, teeth, and oral tissues as clean and sterile as possible by brushing and flossing daily.

Are amalgam fillings safe? Surprisingly, in a large survey with patients, seventy-two percent of the people in the U.S. did not know that amalgam fillings contain about fifty percent mercury. The ADA is careful to only list amalgam fillings as "silver fillings." Mercury has been thought to be a neurotoxin. Studies have shown that up to 27 ug/day of mercury vapor can exude from silver/mercury fillings constantly. Placing amalgam fillings, heavy chewing (bruxism), even rotary cleaning on amalgams can increase the release of mercury vapor. Also, unless trapped, the mercury excess, carved off while filling a tooth goes into the sewer system and eventually down a river or stream, ending up in live fish.

The Scandinavian countries in 2008 banned the use of amalgam fillings in dentistry for the above reasons. The current ADA and FDA position is that amalgams are safe restorative materials. About 35 percent of U. S. dentists still place amalgam fillings. The FDA recently released a new regulation placing amalgam in a "moderate risk" category. I hope people understand what that means. In 2001, the U.S. National Health and nutrition organization surveyed 31,000 adults. They found that the number of dental amalgam fillings correlates to the incidence of heart disease, cancer, mental condition, a thyroid condition, and other neurological problems. However, the Supreme court ruled, "correlation does not demonstrate causation." Only time will tell how much damage, if any, that mercury in fillings will do.

If having mercury fillings removed by a dentist, I suggest you pick an IABDM or IOAMT dentist (check with the ADA or biological dentist). They are trained in the amalgam removal protocol. This is very important. I also suggest that people with cancer have all mercury filling removed.

Also, please do not confuse mercury in amalgam fillings with mercury in pediatric vaccinations. A mercury-based preservative, "thermasol" contains ethyl mercury and is supposed to be nontoxic. Some fish, on the other hand, can contain methyl mercury that is toxic in large amounts.

Some adults with autistic children also suspected that mercury was the causative agent in a large number of autistic children. Dr. Jeffery Bradstreet 6a showed that some vaccinations for these children contained an enzyme called "nagalase." Nagalase blocks the metabolism of vitamin D in a growing child. vitamin D is essential for the development of the brain. With insufficient vitamin D, neurological brain development, and function can be retarded. Unfortunately, Dr. Bradstreet was found dead in a mysterious murder, which they called, suicide. The medical establishment had listed many of these alternative cancer physicians as "Quacks." There is an ongoing feud with the medical establishment. This correlates to 77 alternative cancer and functional medicine doctors who ended up mysteriously dying between 2015 to 2019. 3a This makes a person wonder what is going on!

Fluoride has been put in city drinking water to help reduce cavities since the 1950s. The ADA and the FDA have pushed hard to get fluoride in every city to make teeth harder and prevent cavities. In reality, some natural fluoride may help reduce cavities, but the fluoride that cities put in their water is not natural stream fluoride and is more toxic. A TIME magazine article published in 2010, listed ten common household toxins, including fluoride. It is well known that fluoride can cause thyroid disorders and iodine malabsorption. Fluoride also now comes in toothpaste and mouthwashes. They may not be the best health items to use in the mouth. Toothpaste with hydrogen peroxide and/or baking soda is an alkalizing agent and helps control the bacteria in the mouth. They may not be as sweet but work well. A good sugar-free diet is a great asset.

A great diet, plus a thorough and timely method of brushing (two to four minutes, twice a day), and daily flossing usually cleans teeth thoroughly. This is the best bacteria and toxin reducing habit. Regular visits to the dentist are also a must for keeping healthy teeth.

Another red flag in mouth hygiene starts waving when brushing and flossing are neglected and a person develops bleeding gums. This condition starts very innocently (slight bleeding), but can develop into a gum infection called periodontal disease. That is not good. Not only does brushing neglect start to develop a bad bacterial infestation, but a person starts to lose bone between and around the teeth. Most of these bone loss and periodontal infection people have an acidic body or very low pH. The critical pH of blood, 7.4 is needed to keep the steady rhythm in the heart. In a calcium deficient, (acetic low pH) body, this interdental calcium bone and also calcium from the cervical vertebrae is taken by the blood to raise the blood pH, which moderates the heart rhythm.

You can imagine that as the periodontal infection progresses, dangerous toxins are extruded along with the bleeding, and possible bone loss. As the neglect of brushing and flossing continues, it begins to affect the blood vessels, immune system, body cells, body organs, the heart, and overall health.

A good percentage of young people do not have room for their wisdom teeth. Many of these teeth only erupt one half the way up, are slanted, very crowded, and/or develop pockets that many times create a bacterial infection site. If not straightened or extracted, these wisdom teeth many times create chronic infections that can cause serious problems. The dentist may even feel the lymph nodes in the neck as they become enlarged with the infection. Parents and young adults should be aware of these situations, and in crowded cases, they should either get these teeth straightened or in most cases, when there is no room, extracted. These wisdom teeth infections are another serious problem that can cause inflammation, free radical cell damage, and disease in the body.

That leads to root canals. Did you know that in the past more than fifty percent of the root canals, when finished was not sterile, and when finished, spread toxic bacteria into the blood? Tye Bollinger 9a, author and cancer researcher, from his research with several dentists, oral surgeons, and physicians, states that if you have cancer, you should get all root canal teeth extracted. The reasoning is that teeth have thousands of tiny tubules, each of which needs to be sterilized to have a sterile tooth. Yet with poor sterilization, these teeth can remain infected and harbor testy toxic bacteria for years. After treatment, the bacteria from tubule infections will get back into the blood. The ADA states that these root canal teeth are safe. However, some dental organizations recommend extracting these bacterially infected teeth, rather than choosing a root canal treatment. Recent new sterilization techniques are getting sterile results.

One other oral health problem involves chewing tobacco and smoking. Most teenagers know the dangers of chewing. Every year in the U.S., hundreds of mouth cancers are discovered by dentists, orthodontists, and oral surgeons. A good majority of mouth cancers are caused by chewing tobacco and some from smoking. Thousands of people are admitted to the hospital each year with lung cancer. Tobacco may not be as much of the culprit as the extra nicotine and toxic chemicals, plus the contaminated chemicals in the wrappers. I feel that if a person chews or smokes tobacco, or uses any substitute, he or she should visit the cancer ward of his/her hospital, just to get educated.

There is one other very injurious oral health and medical problem that needs urgent education and better treatment. Most dentists, orthodontists, oral surgeons, neurologists, and back surgeons need to be involved in the body pH, dental bite, temporal mandibular joint, neck muscles, plus knowledge of the cause of scoliosis pressure on the cervical and lumbar vertebrae. Many of these professionals do not understand the connection between a person's abnormal bite, temporal mandibular joint dysfunction, condylar position, the strain on neck muscles, and vertebral malposition with an acetic (low pH), low calcium body.

This situation involves the bite, cervical and lumbar vertebrae. There are over 65 muscles in the neck. A slanted or malaligned occlusion, over closed bite, or accident, resulting in a temporal mandibular dysfunction, can change the head posture of a person. Anterior forward or slanted head posture changes the posterior muscle tension. The change in the head posture puts pressure on the meniscus (cartilage) of the cervical and even the lumbar vertebrae. These vertebral posture changes usually are never detected or related to an abnormal or slanted bite and the pH (acidity) of the body. If we use a pilot's jargon with the bite, we can say that the maxilla and/or bite can have a serious debilitating tilt in three dimensions, or a pitch, roll, or yaw. Pitch meaning a forward posture, either from a slanted (pitch) bite or a bite over closure, temporal mandibular joint over closure, and tightened neck muscles. The forward neck posture causes a cervical vertebrae malalignment due to the posterior neck muscle strain. The vertebral malalignment changes the pressure on the anterior/posterior rims of the cervical vertebrae and meniscus. This is where the acidity of the body (pH) and the blood gets very involved. The uneven vertebral pressure puts undue pressure on the anterior rim of the vertebral cartilages, usually C3, C4, C5, and C6.

In a very acetic body or calcium deficiency, the calcium is usually deficient and the pH is very low. The heart rhythm depends on a constant blood pH to remain at a steady pace. When blood pH gets low, or below 7.35, the blood calls out to the body for calcium to raise the blood to 7.4 pH, and maintain a steady heart rhythm. Osteoclasts, (bone grabbing) calcium molecules in the blood, obtain the calcium from areas of excess pressure, the rim of vertebral cartilages (meniscus), and/or between and around the teeth. There you go, an acidic pH, calcium deficiency, neck muscle tension, slanted bite plus anterior/posterior vertebral pressure causes a cervical vertebral herniation or perforation.

Back surgeons many times needlessly operate on the cervical vertebrae, when the over closed bite, temporal mandibular dysfunction, anterior head posture, posterior neck muscle, and posture strain, plus anterior cervical vertebral pressures are the culprit. Recent research has now shown that posture change can also cause scoliosis and affect lumbar vertebrae. Scoliosis of the lumbar vertebrae can also cause the same cartilage (meniscus) degeneration to occur in acetic bodies. This cartilage robbery process evolves with a herniation or perforation of these vertebral and lumbar cartilages. It has been written that it also can be the cause of a short leg.

That is where the dentists, orthodontists, oral surgeons, neurologists, chiropractors, and back surgeons may be making a mistake. The root of the whole problem starts in the oral cavity and involves the maxilla, TM joint, neck muscles, acidity of the patient, calcium deficiency, blood pH, and the posture. More education needs to be done to inform the dentists, back surgeons, chiropractors, and oral surgeons about this problem. Maybe more TM joint education with doctors involved, communication, knowledgeable TM joint treatment, and posture corrections could save some debilitating cervical and lumbar vertebral cartilage operations. I sure hope this comes about

19

Telomeres: The Secret to Long life

Recently, much research has been done on telomeres and how to keep them from shortening. Telomeres are a nucleotide at the end of each chromosome. They duplicate the DNA and replace aging cells with new cells. As a person ages, telomeres wear down and shorten. New body cells replace the old cells. This process creates new body cells which enhances a person's health and disease resistance associated with aging. The body cells are replenished by the action of the DNA at the end of the telomeres. However, when the cells are replaced, the result is that the telomere ends get shorter.

The shortening of the telomeres is an extension of cell division and aging. Keeping telomeres long is related to fewer cell divisions throughout a person's life. According to researchers, a person has only so many telomere divisions in his or her life. The result is that a person has only so many duplicate body cell changes during their lifetime. Some people say the shortening is related to their genes, but recent research has found that a person's diet, inflammation, and radical body cell damage has a great and damaging influence on telomere shortening. Poor diet, inflammation, leaky gut, and radical body cell damage all cause a faster than normal telomere shortening of one's life. Staying healthy and eating a great diet is related to how long you may live.

Researchers say keeping telomeres longer is related to a hormone called telomerase. Telomerase adds healthy DNA to your chromosomes. They have found that the hormone, telomerase can be enhanced with your diet and some nitric oxide supplements that can keep your telomeres from shortening faster than normal. Poor diet, inflammation, and free radical cell damage all cause a faster than normal telomere shortening which may shorten one's life. When a person boosts his or her telomerase, the telomeres slow down or in some cases, it has been found that the telomeres get longer. Telomerase also adds more

DNA to the chromosomes. This helps prolong a person's energy, heart function, memory, immune system, health, and longevity.

Developing a dynamic diet, plus having a good supplement regime may also be of immense benefit for living a long and healthy life. Dr. David Brownstein 10a has stated that inflammation and free radical body cell damages are the most destructive cause of most diseases and telomere shortening. Intestinal toxins, inflammation, leaky gut, and radical body cell damage can alter the DNA. When DNA gets damaged, it can shorten the telomeres.

Being overweight, eating refined and processed foods, stress, little or no exercise, red meat, sugar, and saturated vegetable oils all create inflammation, radical cell damage, and premature cell death. This damages cell DNA which can shorten the telomeres and a person's life.

The first valuable secret to keeping your telomeres long and happy is by your diet, plus intestinal bacteria in a great 80 – 20 ratio or a good bacteria ratio vs. bad bacteria and with no candida and other parasites.

The following steps are a wise regimen that may contribute to stable telomeres, prevent telomere shortening, have a great immune system, less disease, and longer life. It has been recommended by several leading telomerase treating physicians:

1. Eat a diet that follows the highly nutritious food and supplements in the 54 pages (second section) of this cancer-preventing book. Select and eat the high electromagnetic, nutritional, and neutral pH value foods and supplements.

2. Take 2,000 IU of vitamin D3 every day and/or get 20 minutes of sunshine every day, plus 20 -30 minutes of exercise.

3. Take at least two tablespoons of Omega 3 fatty acids every day*. These can include raw cod liver oil, krill oil, calamari oil, flaxseed oil, avocado oil, Udo's choice, or raw northern seed oils. * very important.

4. Take 500 mg of vitamin C, twice every day. * very important.

5. Get 15-20 minutes of vigorous exercise and take these supplements: L- arginine, turmeric, beetroot powder, Ginkgo

Biloba, and garlic every day. This provides nitric acid which increases body oxygen, an enhancer of long life.

6. Try to take these polyphenols often: blueberries, a small glass of red wine (optional), red grapes, pomegranates, raw red fruits, and raw pears.

7. Get and take two resveratrol tablets every day. Dr. Al Sears and many other telomerase treating physicians say this supplement increases telomerase and keeps telomeres from shortening. A person can get resveratrol from Amazon, Bionutritionals, and/or the Trigen company.

8. Take 12 mg per day of Astaxanthin. Astaxanthin is a powerful antioxidant that attacks inflammation and free cell radicals. My recommendation; Pur Zanthin Ultra from Amazon.

20

Round-Up and GMO Foods, The Nemesis of Health

Genetically modified organisms are where changes are made to the plant DNA to give it resistance to pests and adversaries. In this process, a plant gene can be moved or eliminated, while a gene from another source can be inserted. GMO plants are created to achieve a better yield, a disease-resistant trait, pest-resistant plants, or drought tolerance. But another serious problem exists with a herbicide product, roundup. Supposedly these GMOs and roundup (glyphosate) give farmers protection against specific plant pests and some herbicides. Other advantages are: enhance yield, bigger grains, increase nutritional content, and reduce food waste. There are now about 10-15 different GMO and glyphosate plant crops.

In the U.S., the government and the FDA have excused companies from printing GMO hazard labels, so the consumer usually does not have any way to know which products are GMO added.

Monsanto, who produces Roundup (glyphosate) sells about 300 million gallons every year to spray on crops. It is used on growing vegetable crops, including corn, soy, alfalfa, sorghum, oranges, barley, beets, sugar beets, lemons, Pima cotton, edible beans, apples, papaya, potatoes, many grains, and silage crops. The chemical is sprayed on 89 percent of U.S. corn and 94 percent of soybean crops.

Many other products contain the ingredients from these genetically modified plants. Some of these are sodium ascorbate, vitamin C, citric acid, ethanol, natural flavors, artificial flavorings, fructose, corn syrup, hydrolyzed vegetables, lactic acid, malt dextrin, sodium glutamate (MSG), sucralose, vegetable protein, and xanthan gum.

The body of current EPA and EUc.RfD toxicological studies supporting glyphosate, suggesting that glyphosate, in its pure form, and some glyphosate formulated end-use products may be triggering epigenetic changes through endocrine-mediated mechanisms. Evidence relating to kidney damage, liver, and endocrine changes shows that continued use of glyphosate creates a risk for blood, kidney, and liver damage, plus cancer. More tests need to be carried out to determine the real risks and genetic changes that occur. The EPA has not reported pesticide use data since 2007. That is why over 30 countries have banned GMO products.

The Dewayne Johnson vs. Monsanto lawsuit 7a has brought national attention against Monsanto. The court awarded 289 million dollars to this leukemia patient who is dying. Monsanto has appealed. Mr. Johnson will probably not be around to see the final verdict. Since that lawsuit, more than 4,000 lawsuits have been filed against Monsanto and glyphosate.

To escape the 4,000+ lawsuits and liabilities, Monsanto has been sold to Bayer Aspirin for 66 billion dollars. The Monsanto brand will be discontinued and Bayer will name a new brand, most likely trying to escape new lawsuits. A person can get much more information in a book written by Ocean Robbins, and/or the Food Revolution Network. Their address is P.O. Box 3563, Santa Cruz, CA. 95053. Also, much more information about GMO foods can be obtained on the computer. My advice is to buy organic foods as much as possible and try to limit refined and processed foods with corn and soy unless they are organic.

Biology professor Michael Skinner 8a at Washington State University studied the effects of glyphosate in rats. He exposed pregnant rats to glyphosate. The rats had no harmful side effects. The rat's children were also OK with no genetic effects. The grandchildren also were okay. However, more than 90 percent of the great-grandchildren developed one or more diseases. The diseases ran from tumors of the prostate to major birth defects. Skinner said that the glyphosate changes the epigenetics in the sperm and/or eggs of the individual exposed to the glyphosate. The genetic traits are passed on to the next generation and it keeps going for generations to come. Skinner said that the administration of the chemical was a standard approach.

Skinner's tests were disputed by Bill Reeves, a toxicologist with Monsanto/Bayer. Skinner argued that the tests Reeves made were flawed. They did not represent the administration of the chemical because the rats were injected in the abdomen in the Reeves study. Skinner said that it is not the way that humans would be exposed to glyphosate. The study was peer-reviewed and published in an accredited scientific journal. Skinner also said that the tumors occurred because of an epigenetic shift in the sperm or egg of the first generation of the pregnant rats. That it was passed on by a generational genetic effect.

21

If You Have Cancer.
Why You Need to Ask Some Very
Critical Questions

A very critical question is how to treat your cancer? It may be the difference between life and death. First of all, you need to be sure your diagnosis is correct. You may want a second or third opinion. Is your tumor a fast or slow-growing cancer? You may also want to get two or three options or opinions on how to treat it.

For example, with prostate cancer, there are four or five different ways it can be treated. However, many oncologists who favor surgery may not explain what the results of surgery will be or explain the other ways prostate cancer can be treated. They may not tell you that surgery may make you sterile, you may not be able to get an erection, plus there may be incontinence with urine dripping and even sometimes bowel elimination problems. Also, new alternative techniques, the VIPP thearpy machine and the 4-in-1 blanket, drugs, and proton radiation are improving, making successful cure a realization. Most prostate surgeries end up with incontinence.

Your decision for treatment is very important. It is wise to study your treatment choices with your family, naturopath, physician, and oncologist.

I have compiled some very important questions that you can ask your physician and oncologist. It may not be a complete list. Use what you like. You may think of others that are related to your cancer. Don't be afraid to ask any questions that you feel are pertinent to your treatment. It may be wise to copy any of these questions on a separate sheet and leave room for you to put down the answers.

The answers will be of great value as to your decision on the knowledge and treatment by the physician and/or oncologist. They may also be important in your decision to use conventional treatment, combinations of treatment, find an alternative cancer clinic, or consult with a treatment facility.

These questions will help you decide with your family the type of treatment that you wish to follow. Answers to many of these may also help you make logical decisions about your treatment.

A suggested list of questions is as follows:

1. What kind of cancer do I have?

2. Is it fast or slow-growing cancer?

3. How much time do I have to decide what course to follow?

4. What do you think is the reason I got this cancer?

5. What are your treatment recommendations?

6. Do you have a diet recommendation to go along with your treatment?

7. Are there any drugs that you will be using?

8. What are the immediate and long term effects of any drugs?

9. Will any of these drugs cause secondary effects or cancer?

10. Will your treatment cure my cancer or just get rid of the symptoms?

11. Will your treatment kill the regular cancer cells and also the stem cells?

12. What is the five-year survival rate for treating my kind of cancer?

13. How long will I have if I do not have any treatment?

14. If you use surgery, chemotherapy, or radiation, what are the short term, and long term effects of treatment?

15. Have you any research studies on the effects or success of the drugs you are using?

16. Can I get a list from you of the drugs you will be using?

17. Can I get a list from you on what steps I need to take with my diet, lifestyle, exercise, foods to avoid, and other vital considerations?

18. Should I take antibiotics if I need them during treatment?

19. I have read that if I have cancer, I will need to stop all sugar, sugar products, most carbohydrates, preservatives, red meat, and all vegetable oils on the grocery shelf. What are your recommendations?

20. Will you be testing my urine or blood with a cancer test? I read that it is mandatory in Greece and will show which drugs work best with my cancer?

21. Is there any toxicity test that may find out if I have toxicity to any of the drugs you will use?

22. What is your cancer cure rate for the patients you have treated with my type of cancer?

23. Do you have a ballpark cost on the type of treatment you are recommending?

24. Is it possible that my body can cure this cancer with alternative treatment?

25. If I decide to do only part of my treatment, will you still be my physician?

26. What supplements will you recommend for my type of cancer?

27. Is it true that cancer is an oxygen deprivation disease and that oxygen therapy, exercise, or hyperbaric oxygen will help?

28. Would you recommend any amino acids or pancreatic enzymes that might help me?

29. What information can I get from you today which will help me decide what I should do?

30. I read that some new treatments are available today which treat my cancer. Do you know what they are?

31. What treatment would you use if you or your wife developed my type of cancer?

32. Thank you for your patience, expertise, and knowledge.

22

Critical Life Saving Treatment for Cancer Victims

If you have cancer, or if you want to prevent cancer, this section lists many, but not all, of the critical alternative treatment modalities used by more than five alternative doctors including Drs. Gonzalez, Kelley, Pauling, Budwig, Beard, Gerson, Michael Cutler, and others included in Suzanne Somer's book. Remember that alternative cancer treatment will cure many but not all cancers. Recent research has shown that chemotherapy and radiation in hundreds of cancer patients can be reduced significantly with these procedures, plus using Johanna Budwig's cottage cheese/flaxseed/kefir/crushed flaxseed formula, every day. Some oncologists may say this is nonsense. Do not believe them. According to Dr. Otto Warburg and others, you need oxygen, detoxification, pancreatic enzymes, etc. You get help from live electromagnetic foods and juices, coffee enemas, pancreatic enzymes, vitamin C, ozone, H2O2 plus many other supplements on the following pages. Most oncologists will not recognize this in addition to their treatment.

If you have decided to have conventional treatment, you may want to explain to the oncologist that you would like to follow the diet, enzyme, supplement, and detoxification therapies along with chemo and/or radiation. You may want to choose some alternative modalities with conventional treatment.

One option is to use the oncologist's full procedures. The second option, you can use conventional along with the other options, like I.V. Vitamin C therapy. The third option, communicate with and use one of the alternative cancer clinics mentioned in this book. The fourth option, if you choose and follow the alternative procedures, you must follow the procedures 100 percent. The fifth option, if you have prostate or breast cancer, proton therapy, or CellSonic electrohydraulic therapy. Remember, there are several books listed that you can get.

If you are having full or partial oncologist treatment, these book treatment options may also be added and be very critical and necessary to save your life. It will help you continue to keep cancer away. Remember that if you decide to treat your cancer without a conventional oncologist's treatment, it is still essential to consult with a cancer physician or alternative cancer physician and listen to his or her advice plus use all of the recommended procedures below. They will have other procedures that you may need. Your computer can also get you in touch with all of the excellent clinics and information for the physicians listed in the book.

This book lists only some very essential critical clinics and books. This information should not be considered as a complete source or sure cancer cure. The information also will not cure all cancers. Recently, many new products and techniques have been introduced. Keep up with all of the new procedures on the internet.

Two books That I suggest you get:

"Victory Over Cancer" http://www.drkelley.info 623 327 1778.

"How to Cure Almost Any Cancer and Natural Cancer Remedies" Online Publishing and Marketing, LLC. P.O. 1076 Lexington, VA. 24450,

The following pages are very critical and essential if you choose an alternative treatment. Skipping any part will leave you more likely to have a failure. Your life will depend on it. Cancer may kill you if you do nothing yourself.

Necessary Mandatory Cancer Procedures

Procedures will say critical and very critical. This is very essential and should be reduced when cancer is gone but prevention continued for life

1. a. Critical: Dr. Joanna Budwig made some of the most essential cancer-curing discoveries of all time. You can read

about these discoveries in chapter 33. She was a biochemist and physicist who discovered under the microscope that all cancer patients had greenish-red blood cells that were colored because of coagulated (sticky homocysteine) blood. She then discovered a food mixture that would unravel sticky blood in cancer patients. If you have cancer, or if you want to prevent cancer, you need to read chapter 33. It is essential.

b. Eat 7-11 fresh, raw vegetables, and raw fruits, nuts, berries, melons, squash, and leaves every day AND/OR 2-4 glasses of raw fresh vegetables and fruit juice with a lemon every day. Make in a juicer.

c. Get an ozone machine. You can even sleep with windows open if possible. d. Try to get 15 minutes of sun every day, plus Vit. D3, 20,000 -25,000 IU. e. Drink lemon juice before bedtime and in the morning when getting up. (critical) Use four tablespoons of raw, fresh pure lemon juice in a glass of water.

2. Toxin removal: (very critical) COFFEE ENEMAS. Get a Gerson coffee enema set on the computer or from amazon. 1. With cancer, one or two coffee enemas every day. 2. Get okra pepsin E-3, from Standard Process. Call Standard Process and find the name of their closest distributor. Take every day for 3 weeks, then renew dosages every 2 months. (critical).

3. Pancreatic Enzymes: (very critical) There are two kinds of pancreatic enzymes. If you have cancer, you must take ONE OR THE OTHER. Rx: Take for 2-4 months, possibly more.

a. Solozyme enzymes. 360 counts, $250.00. Take 12 – 20 tabs a day between meals. Do not eat after 3:00 PM

b. Solozyme enzymes have more pancreatin than Wobenzym–N and are more efficient. Solozyme enzymes are the enzymes that Dr. Gonzalez and Dr. Kelley used to help cure over 20,000 cancer patients. Solozyme enzymes are obtained from www.collegehealthstoreses.com, 817 458 9241.

c. Dr. Kelley's enzymes are the # 1 cancer eradicator. Rx: A person needs 12 – 20 tablets a day, between meals. Continue for two to three months, maybe longer if the cancer isn't gone. Your life may depend on it. (very critical). Dr. Kelley said that these enzymes were very critical in saving his life when he had pancreatic cancer. He also saved the lives of over 10,000 cancer patients. His son, John, now has the formulation.

4. Wobenzym - N enzymes: Obtained from Garden of Life, 4200 Northcorp Parkway, Palm Beach Garden, Fl., 33410. Amazon or online. www.gardenoflife.com. With cancer, a person needs 12-20 tablets each day between meals. (very critical), if you can't get Solozyme enzymes.

5. Peptides: Peptides will help along with enzymes. Get directions from the dealer. Get from: New England Peptides, 1 800 343 5974. (critical).

6. Diet: Live electromagnetic food only. (critical).

1. Eggs; 4 – 6 eggs a week, slightly boiled or raw.

2. Fermented foods: Eat some fermented foods such as kimchi, sauerkraut, beets, kombucha, etc. each day.

3. 4 oz. only of fish or chicken if wanted, every other day.

4. Legumes, lentils, beans, peas, etc. Good in soups.

5. Green tea, other teas.

6. Plain yogurt, cottage cheese.

7. Moderate to small portions of all foods in electromagnetic book section II, categories 10 through 7.

8. Do not eat anything after 3:00 pm.

9. Take iodine every day.

10. Raw nuts: almonds, pecans, walnuts. 4 of each daily,

11. Barley power if acidic, can put in soups, other foods.

7. Critical Supplements needed:

   1. L-arginine

   2. Turmeric

   3. Vitamin D3, 20,000 t0 25,000 IU/day. (sunshine).

   4. Folic acid, B6, B12.

   5. CoQ10

   6. Ginko Biloba.

   7. Vit. C, 4,000- 6000mg. mg. vitamin C/day.

   8. Resveratrol.

   9. Laetrile, from apricot seeds Get from www. cytopharmaonline.com. 1 888 271 4184 or from www. apricotpower.com.

   10. L – lysine.

   11. Iodine.

   12. Beta 1-3 D Glucan, www.ancient5.com 1 855 877 8220, One tablet daily. (crucial).

   13. Hemp Oil, one teaspoon raw hemp oil daily.

   14. Barley powder is essential for acidic bodies. You can use it for an alkalizing agent, 6– 10 tabs daily, if you have an acetic pH.

   15. Greene Supreme, (to raise alkalinity) 1 724 946 9057. Keep checking to stay in the 6.4 to 7.0 pH range.

   16. Iodine. I know this is a lot, but when you have cancer, your life depends on it.

8. Decrease body toxins: (critical)

   a. Get rid of all amalgam in fillings.

b. Do not cook on aluminum cookware.

c. Take frequent hot baths, use the sauna or hot tub.

d. Drink no tap water or water in plastic bottles. Distilled water best.

e. Do not use plastic or aluminum wrap.

Things to Avoid in Cancer Treatment:
All of these are very critical

1. Stop all non-electromagnetic (dead) foods.

2. No sugar, sugar products, sugar substitutes.

3. Stop all vegetable oils, deep-fried, fried foods.

4. No processed or refined foods.

5. No lectins (peanuts, cashews, tomatoes, potatoes).

6. No red meat, sausage, wieners, bacon, etc.

7. No pasteurized milk, cream, ice cream, shakes.

8. Stop all GMO foods.

9. Stop all microwaved foods. Heat in Oven.

10. Limit alcoholic drinks to champagne and beer.

11. No plain or diet sodas.

Notice: Smaller dosages of chemo and radiation may be used with these procedures if you use this regimen and it is approved by your oncologist.

Get rid of all stress. Praise and thank God for this discovery and your life. He will be with you and help you.

William Kelley treated Steve McQueen. McQueen would have gotten better if he had followed Dr. Kelley's advice, but he didn't. You can only win if you follow these complete directions listed on these treatment pages. Be sure that your cancer physician is advised and working with you.

Advice for PREVENTING cancer For those who wish to PREVENT cancer, the directions above can be applied for you with these changes. A. With the pancreatic enzymes, Wobenzym-N is a lot cheaper than Solozyme enzymes, but not quite as good. They contain some very good enzymes that are needed to prevent cancer. For preventing cancer, please reduce the full amount and take 2-3 tablets/day of Solozymes or Wobenzym–N. This prevention is after cancer cure.

1. Coffee enemas may be reduced to one enema a month.

2. Okra pepsin is good and can be used once per year.

3. Fresh raw vegetable and fruit juices are still important and a person could juice and drink up to 1-2 glasses/day.

4. All supplements listed are very good for preventing cancer.

5. Oxygen is very critical for everyone. Use exercise and as many ways as possible to ensure that you get plenty of oxygen. Remember, lack of body cell oxygen is a major cause of cancer. Try to get: Intense or moderate exercise, 15+ minutes per day.

6. All foods: Stay with foods in the book's second section labeled 10 -7 (electromagnetic and nutrition rating, top left).

Cancer advice:

1. You can get some preventive cancer and cancer treatment advice as stated by Dr. William Kelley, Dr. David Brownfield, and Dr. Gonzalez, on the computer.

a. Reduce radiation damage: X-rays, cat scans.

b. Get tested for elevated body metals, parasites, iodine, (critical for cancer patients), vitamins, nutrients, plus hair analysis.

c. It is now known that sugars, red meat, refined foods, carbohydrates, candida, and dead vegetable oils are the direct cause of most people's arthritis, HBP, and cancer.

d. GMO foods are now in 30,000 products.

e. Greatly reduce or eat no sugar, preservatives, artificial sweeteners, diet pop, reduce all carbs, including breakfast cereals, reduce bread (only rye), pasta, milk, no white table salt (use Himalayan salt). no (dead) vegetable oils on the grocery shelf, no refined foods, and no statin drugs. Get only organic foods.

Be sure to look on the computer: http://www.drkelley.info themetabolicdr@aol.com Nicholas Gonzalez Foundation. email: ngonzalezoffice@gmail.com, GonzalezProtocol.com, and please order Dr. Kelley's, Victory Over Cancer, and Dr. Gonzalez's book, One Man Alone, plus Dr. Brownfield's books.

Other notes: Dr. Otto Warburg found that the fermentation without oxygen in cancer cells leads to acidosis and more cancer cells. Linus Pauling found that I.V. therapy with vitamin C (ascorbate) was a very good cancer cell destroyer, and neutralizes acidosis, which is very critical in destroying cancer cells.

Recently, the use of Dr. Pauling's treatment, Less Chemo with I.V. Vitamin C therapy has gotten a very popular rebound in cancer treatment. Ascorbate will counteract the cancer acidosis and create H_2O_2 where the mitochondria generate oxygen which helps kill the cancer cells. It is a very successful adjunct that can be used with chemotherapy. Doctors are using smaller dosages of Chemo with I.V. ascorbate and iron, which is a great help in killing the cancer stem cells and creates a more successful result.

If you have any questions about the use of I.V. vitamin C (ascorbate) therapy for cancer you might contact the RIORDAN CLINIC or Dr. Ron Hunninghake. Their phone number is 1 800 447 7276.

Good News about Treating Some Cancers

Treating B-cell lymphoblastic leukemia, multiple myeloma, and non-Hodgkin's lymphoma. There is a new technique of cancer treatment called CAR-T therapy, TCR, and CRISPR-Cas9 using drugs made by the Calgene Drug Company. CRISPR is an advancement of genetic cell editing technology. Genetic editing allows the body to "cut" mutated parts of the cell DNA (diribonucleic acid) or "cut and replace" segments of DNA that contain mutated cancer cells.

The action of CRISPR: It targets genetic mutations in the body and "edits" out the mutations without hardly any side effects. The technique uses what is called CAR-T therapy. It has been very successful in treating B-cell acute lymphoblastic leukemia, non-Hodgkin's lymphoma, and multiple myeloma without side effects. Trials have shown that there is an 85 percent complete remission rate within three months of treatment. The treatment has very little discomfort for the patient.

These results are real and no longer a speculation. The technique by the Calgene Company is now being tested on solid tumors with good results. If you are diagnosed with any one of these tumors you need to consult with your oncologist before trying this treatment.

Hemp Research: Although cancer cells use multiple mechanisms to evade immune responses, the development of these hemp immune therapeutic approaches may assist in the future in eliminating cancer tumors. Companies are now researching the developing use of hemp (cannabinoid) varieties in treating some forms of cancer. Keep up on these products (keep up on Google and other research applications) because there is a lot of new research by many companies. Pascal Biosciences in Seattle is one of those firms that is making great strides in curing some malignancies with cannabinoids. Check about Cannabis with your Functional Medicine Physician.

The HCG Urine cancer test, how to test for cancer: A \$55.00 cancer test to see if you have gotten rid of cancer or still have it. (human chorionic gonadotropin test). Score: If it is 50 or more you have cancer. If the score is 49 or less, you have only the normal amount of cancer hits.

1. Get an early morning urine sample.

2. Take 50 CC, (2 oz) out.

3. Add 200 cc. acetone and 5 ccs. of ethyl or methyl alcohol.

4. Stir.

5. Let stand in the refrigerator for 6 – 8 hours.

6. There should be sediment on the bottom. Remove one half of the top (clear) solution. Leave bottom ½ with sediment. Filter the rest of the solution with sediment in a coffee filter.

7. After filtration, DRY filter with sediment, fold and put in the plastic bag.

8. Send by the fastest air carrier to Navarro Medical Clinic, Dr. Efren Navarro, 3553 Signing Street, Morningside Terrace, Santa Mesa, Manila 1016, Philippines.

9. Get a $55.00 cashier's check, make a copy, and send it with the sample to Mrs. Erlinda Suarez with the patient's name, address, sex, age, and a brief clinical history or diagnosis. Include your email address. Do not send the check to Dr. Navarro. 10. Send the $55.00 cashier's check or money order to Mrs. Erlinda Suarez, 631 peregrine Drive, Palatine, IL. 60067. Dr. Navarro's phone number is 011 632 714 7442

23

Important Alternative Cancer clinics

If you wish to use an alternative cancer clinic, these are a few of the recommended clinics in the US. and elsewhere.

1. The Gonzalez clinic, New York. www.dr-gonzalez.com Information also can be found on the computer. 1 212 213 3337

2. The Gerson clinic, Chipsa Hospital, Nubes 670 Esquina Creston. Secc.jar Del Sol, Playas Tijuana, Baja California 22505 Mexico CityCP 1 888 667 3640 1 855 624 4772

3. Very good German clinics.www. germanCancerBreakthrough.com

4. Dr. John Lubecki's clinic, Fair Oaks, California.www. Lubecki-Chiropractic.com

5. The Budwig clinic, Callo Rio Mesa 28, Floor 1 office. Torremolinos, 129620, Malaga, Spain Phone: 1 866 251 3569 www.contact@budwigcenter.com www.joannabudwig. com 34 952 577 369

6. Calgary Centre for Naturopathic Medicine, Calgary, Alberta, Canada www.CalgaryNaturopathic.com

7. Dr. Frank Cousineau. www.Adios-Cancer.com

8. The University of Loma Linda Cancer Hospital. 1-800-protons 1 888 317 0793

9. California, Loma Linda Proton Beam Cancer Center. www.protons.com

24

Vaccines, Autism, and Vanishing Alternative Cancer Doctors

In 2018 the FDA approved VAXELIS, a six in one children's combo vaccine produced by Merck and Sanofi. The vaccine claims that it will prevent diphtheria, tetanus, pertussis, poliomyelitis, and type B influenza.

"The Truth About Cancer," an organization originated by Tye Bollinger, 9a has written a rebuttal that may be very interesting to most people. It is entitled, "FDA approves VAXELIS combo vaccine despite a short duration of studies and tests." While most drug studies last for months or even years, vaccines are evaluated for a far lesser time. According to Ty Bollinger, there's evidence that the preservatives in this vaccine, like aluminum and mercury, may be related to the alarming rise in AUTISM across America. The duration of the studies with this vaccine was much smaller than any other drug-seeking FDA approval.

Merck is one of the biggest vaccine manufacturers in the U.S. and has been involved in several lawsuits, alleging misconduct, falsifying research information, plus influencing government oversite. The CDC's claim that vaccines do not cause autism is largely based on one study conducted in 2004, overseen by a senior scientist, William Thompson. In 2014 Thompson confessed that the agency actively destroyed any data linking Merck's MMR vaccine to autism, stating that "the omitted data suggested that African American males who received MMR vaccine before age 36 months were at a greater risk for autism."

The HPV vaccine has more documented cases of adverse reactions than any other vaccine in the world. However, it is still administered in the U.S. Please do not think that I am against the VAXELIS OR OTHER VACCINES. I just think every health professional and citizen should spend time learning about the vaccines given to children. All children need to be vaccinated.

There were mysterious deaths of more than seventy-seven alternative cancer and autism treatment doctors between 2015 and 2019: Dr. NICKOLAS GONZALEZ was one of the more than seventy-seven alternative autism and cancer practitioners who have mysteriously died in those years. Dr. Gonzalez was only 64 years old and in great health. Regardless of what the ADA says, his clinic had treated over 10,000 cancer patients, with a very successful cure rate of over 75 percent, even with grade 3 and 4 cancer patients. It does not correspond that during this time, not one oncologist who treats cancer with the regular treatment of chemo, drugs, and radiation, has mysteriously died Some of Dr. Gonzalez's treatment is described in this book. More information can be found by checking his website and by reading his book, "One Man Alone." One Man Alone is a book about a dentist, Dr. William Kelley, who had pancreatic cancer and was given four months to live after having chemotherapy and radiation treatment. Dr. Kelley cured his cancer and went on to cure many more thousands of cancer patients. Dr. Gonzalez has also written many other books that are of great value to anyone who wants to prevent cancer or who has cancer. However, the medical establishment gives him a bad rap on his website, although he has had a much better average ratio of success treating cancer than the medical establishment.

The modern standard treatment of cancer using chemotherapy, drugs. and radiation by most oncologists has not changed for over 60 years. The cancer success result has not changed much for that same period. The treatment is mostly directed toward cancer symptom treatment, and most of the time does not get rid of the stem cells in many cancers. Cancer has two types of cells, regular and stem cells. Both types need to be eradicated for the cure of cancer. Cancer treatment costs, paid by insurance companies and from patients in the U. S., is about 180 to 200 billion dollars per year.

The mysterious death of Dr. JEFFERY BRADSTREET: 6a Dr. Bradstreet treated autism and cancer with a globulin component macrophage activating factor called GcMAF. It is a glycosylated vitamin D binding regulatory protein normally present in the immune system. It is found in healthy individuals but lacking in people with autism and cancer. It has been shown to improve immune system function. Dr. Bradstreet had treated over 11,000 autism and cancer patients with a much better than normal autism and cancer treatment result. Three days after the FDA raided his office and laboratory, Dr. Bradstreet was found dead, shot in the chest, floating down a nearby river.

There are over seventy-five more mysterious alternative autism and cancer doctor death stories that can and should be told. Maybe someday it will all be unraveled.

About GcMAF: GcMAF activation in the body can be an important prevention immune response. GcMAF activates macrophages, which are white blood cells that digest cellular debris, foreign substances, bacteria, cancer, and other cells. When GcMAF is low or depleted, the body's immune response and macrophage activity become weak.

Vitamin D is important in the development and maintenance of the central nervous system. It is essential for babies and is critical during pregnancy. It is required for emotional and cognitive thought plus the development of new brain cells. It also is very valuable in preventing coronavirus.

A vitamin D deficiency can disrupt the proper development of the brain and immune system while affecting the brain and spinal cord. Dr. Bradstreet's therapy using both Vitamin D and GcMAF enhanced the immune system and helping most autism patients get much improved.

Nagalase enzyme is produced by viruses, cancer cells, and bacteria. It inhibits macrophage immune production and vitality. Tye Bollinger, in his criticism of the preservatives in vaccines, may have been referring to the production of nagalase, which is counterproductive and harmful in both autism and cancer. Dr. Bradstreet found that injecting GcMAF decreases nagalase, reduces cancer tumors, and eradicates many types of cancers.

Certain supplements help GcMAF do its job. These are vitamins D3, oleic acid (extra virgin olive oil), and avocados. Even to prevent cancer, these supplements are a vital adjunct to your immune system. Vitamin D3 recommendation is 10.000 to 20,000 IU. With cancer, 20,000 to 25,000 IU.

A medical organization in Japan called; Saiei Mirai, manufacturers, and has tested an injectable form of GcMAF along with bovine colostrum products. These products can be purchased from their website. Colostrum has been shown to activate GcMAF. (http://saisei-mirai.or.jp/macrophage_eng.html) "Bravo Yogurt" and GcMAF: There is also a yogurt that activates GcMAF. It is called "Bravo Yogurt." Dr. John Gray, on his website (MarsVenus.com), describes Bravo Yogurt as having 42 essential probiotics to restore healthy gut function and production of GcMAF. Dr. Gray, the man who wrote "Men are from Mars, Women are from Venus," has a lot of advice on the brain, and brain function.

25

Where to Obtain Your Cancer Regimen

The following is a long list, but you are dealing with your life. These foods, supplements, formulas, tests, and supplies are worth the time, money, and effort. For prevention, you will want to take reduced amounts of supplies and supplements.

1. Joanna Budwig's critical formula, listed in Chapter 33, is a life-saving cottage cheese/flaxseed oil/quark/crushed flaxseed mixture. This formula is essential for every cancer patient. Without this formula, most cancer patients would not receive enough oxygen and free blood to cure cancer. You can read her critical discoveries about coagulated (sticky) blood and the cottage cheese/flaxseed formula, and how she cured grade 3 and grade 4 cancer in patients who had been given two weeks to two months to live after chemotherapy and radiation treatment. With her formula, she had a 75 to 85% recovery with these patients. See chapter 33.

2. Wobenzym-N, Garden of Life, 4299 Northcorp Parkway, Palm Beach Garden, Fl. 33410. Get online, 800 tabs. For cancer, take 12-18 per day between meals. For prevention, take 3 tabs daily. Remember, solozyme enzymes have more pancreatin and are more effective.

3. Solozyme enzymes, www.collegehealthstores.com. 817458 9241. 12-18 tabs each day between meals.

4. Barley powder, (to raise alkalinity). Get from Greene supreme, Inc. 200, and 400 tablet bottles. For cancer, if acidic, 15 tabs a day between meals. Check pH twice daily. If over 6.8, stop powder. Keep the neutral pH. Preventive dose 2-4 tabs daily. 1 724 946 9057, or 1 800 358 0777.

5. Vit. D3, From Daily manufacturing, 4820 Pless road, Rockwell, N.C. 28138, 1 800 868 0700, www.dailymfg.com, 20,00-25,000IU daily. less for prevention.

6. Beta-1 - 3 D Glucan, (Enhances neutrophils which kill cancer cells) 500 mg tablets, www.ancient5.com. 1 855 877 8220, take 3 tabs daily.

7. Vitamin C, (Spectra-Scorb Plus, time-release) 1000 mg tabs. For cancer take 3 tabs, every 12 hours. For prevention, 2 tabs 24 hours apart. Get from Daily Mfg. 1 800 868 0700 (see above).

8. pH paper, From Daily Mfg. (above) or Green Supreme, 1 724 946 9057. or online. You should get pH rolls that read, from 4.5 to 8 or 9.

9. Iodine, vitamins, and minerals, most can be gotten from Daily Manufacturing. 1 800 868 0700. Take the required amounts listed daily.

10. L-Proline, L-Lysine, (combination). (inhibits metastasis of cancer cells), 500 mg. tabs, Take 2 tabs daily. Get online, Pro Rite or others, or on Amazon.

11. Cell Forte, (enzyme therapy) (Max 3w/w miatake and cats claw), 120 caps, 1 800 783 2286. 500 mg tabs, take 2 tabs twice daily.

12. Avemar, (Helps stop cancer from using glucose), American Biosciences www.americanbiosciences.com, 1 888 884 7700, oral dosage, 8.5 gms for 150 lb. person.

13. Laetrile, (from apricot seeds), You can get laetrile at 1 888 271 4184 www.cytopharmaonline.com, or www.cancerchoices.com. 5 tabs daily.

14. Immune Assist: Aloha Medicinals or online. www.alohamedicinals.com 500 mg tabs, 2 tabs daily.

15. Transfer Factor Plus, Aloha Medicinals (above) 500 to 960 mg tabs, take 2 tabs daily.

16. Coffee enema set, order the Gerson coffee enema set, Amazon

17. Dr. Navarro cancer test kit, (All the supplies for performing the cancer test on life-saving treatments chapter). The kit provides acetone, other supplies, instructions, and everything you need to prepare the urine for shipment. www. JoeBallCompany.com Dr. Navarro's (the cancer urine test) phone no. is 011 632 714 7442. You can get the cancer test and sending the dried urine sample to Dr. Navarro's clinic in the Philippines. See chapter 22; (Critical life-saving treatment for cancer victims)

18. Green tea, Essiac, and Pau D'arco tea, these teas fight both inflammation and cancer. They are all highly recommended for prevention and helping to cure cancer. Your computer has a lot of information on these products. You can order Pau D'arco tea bark from your local health store. Ask the manager to special order it if it is not in stock.

If you have any questions about these supplies, supplements, preventing or helping to cure cancer, you can call me at 1 509 670 2490, or email me at DrMEL11@aol.com. I will try to answer all questions.

26

Dr. Joanna Budwig and
Her Incredible Cancer Discoveries

Dr. Joanna Budwig made some of the greatest essential cancer discoveries of all time. She was a biochemist and physicist who found some severe discrepancies in the red blood cells of cancer patients. Her amazing discoveries followed Dr. Otto Warburg and Linus Pauling's great work. Her cancer interests led her to examine the red blood cells of cancer patients under the microscope.

Dr. Budwig's blood discoveries began with her microscope evaluation of the blood in cancer patients. She was the first person to devise a chemical measurement to test red blood fat metabolism. She devised a technique to analyze a cancer patient's blood. What she found was a revelation in cancer research. Her new technology soon became a routine used around the world.

Dr. Budwig found that the blood in a cancer patient had a strange greenish color. She found that the color came from platelet coagulation (sticky blood). Her analysis then led her to find that almost every cancer patient's blood was carrying very little oxygen. The coagulation or sticky (homocysteine) blood was keeping the red blood cells from carrying oxygen. The result was that the body and organ cells were being starved of oxygen. This situation was weakening the body cells and the immune system. The cancer cells love no oxygen since they multiply and metastasize with a process of glucose metabolism or glycation. From her biochemistry and physicist knowledge, and examining further, Budwig found that the cause of the oxygen starvation in a cancer patient's blood came from an excess of omega 6 fatty acids (vegetable oils on the grocery shelf), plus an acidic body. These fatty acids form "transfats and mega trans" which came from the partially hydrogenated oils in their diet. Since these oils have no electromagnetic charge, they are dead oils and cause a reaction with cancer cell toxins in the blood which restricts the oxygen. The transfats and mega trans which were changing the composition of the blood are the same as those oils found on the grocery shelf, which have been boiled to prevent them from being rancid. Boiling takes the electromagnetism out of the oils, unlike the cold-pressed electromagnetic oils that are in the molecules of polyunsaturated and monounsaturated COLD PRESSED oils. The non-electromagnetic oils are responsible for forming the coagulated, (sticky) greenish blood that carries no oxygen in cancer patients. The non-electromagnetic oils on the grocery shelf also are the culprits that cause coagulation (sticky blood) in other diseases. They are connected with high blood pressure, heart disease, strokes, heart attacks, and some diabetes. The body cell oxygen starvation paves the way for cancer cells to multiply and metastasize since they need no oxygen. They use sugar, sugar products, carbohydrates, and protein to propagate.

Dr. Budwig's incredible discoveries establishedseveral very critical and important cancer facts:

1. Almost all cancer patients have blood with a greenish color which comes from coagulated (sticky) red blood cells that carry little or no oxygen.

2. The oxygen starvation of the body cells weakens the whole body and the immune system. This allows cancer cells to multiply and thrive.

3. Cancer cells love little or no oxygen.

4. The first line of defense for treating cancer should be to unravel the coagulated (sticky) blood.

5. The first thing every oncologist should do is to inform every cancer patient right away from this important discovery. They very seldom do.

6. If you, your relative, or your neighbor has cancer, it would be wise to inform them of Dr. Budwig's oxygen starvation and unraveling technique which will be discussed below.

Dr. Budwig's second evolutionary discovery was a food mixture she found that would unravel the greenish coagulated (sticky) blood. Her mixture would unravel the red blood cells, enabling them to carry oxygen to the body cells and organs. This strengthens the body cells and the immune system, which is direly needed to cure cancer.

Dr. Budwig found, that when she mixed cottage cheese, cold raw flaxseed oil, crushed raw flaxseeds, and Quark, which is like plain kefir, except it can produce a reaction of the sulphydryl groups, allowing the flaxseeds to become water- soluble. Kifer will not be as effective in this reaction. That is why it is better to use Quark, if possible kefir should not be used. In the U.S., a person needs to order Quark from the health food store. It is called "Nancy's organic Quark." If it is not available, ask if you can order it.

Dr. Budwig got 100 patients from her local hospital and tested her formula. She also used many other kinds of treatments with her cottage cheese/flaxseed.

27

A Great New Paradigm of Health Treatment

We are living in the greatest era in medical history. However, the medical establishment in the U.S. is holding back on some great alternative treatments that are saving about 75 to 85 percent of cancer patients in other countries. How long this situation will go on depends on changes by the FDA, drug companies, and the U.S. government. The situation in blocking new alternative treatments for cancer impedes some very effective cancer cures.

Many foreign nations are using great, new cancer-fighting instruments, new diets, detoxification, and other methods that are now being subdued by the U.S. medical establishment. Most nations are allowed to use whatever treatment that works best for their cancer patients. Some nations use small doses of chemo, radiation, and chemo drugs, along with I. V. vitamin C, enzymes, coffee enemas, diet changes, food restrictions, I.V. Mistletoe, and other I.V. treatments. Many do not use chemotherapy, chemo drugs, and radiation at all. Others use electrical impulse (vibrations) instruments along with the above-mentioned therapies. In almost all cases, other country cancer physicians will use changes in the diet, liver detoxification, infrared saunas, fresh raw plant foods, nuts, enzymes, raw, and fresh vegetable juices with lemon. They also restrict sugars, sugar substances, preservatives, refined and processed carbohydrates, omega 6 vegetable oils, red meat, and many other foods.

Recently, newer cancer instruments are being used in many countries that help cure cancer. One instrument that is being used with remarkable success is the CellSonic electro-hydraulic VIPP therapy instrument. Doctors in Mexico, Spain, India, Germany, Peru, and other countries are very pleased with the non-invasive cancer cell destroying results. The CellSonic therapy instrument works by sending a high voltage electrical pulse (vibration) into the cancer area. The electrical impulse alters the polarity of the cancer cells. This creates changes in the mutated cancer cells that change them back into normal body cell polarity.

The CellSonic therapy instrument does many other remarkable disease transformations and cures. With the intense pressure shockwave pulse, the instrument produces exceptional success in many diseases and ailments. These include gallstones, kidney stones, sports injuries, wound healing, rheumatic arthritis, migraine headaches, enlarged prostate, stenosis, avascular neuritis, diabetes, and many other diseases and ailments. The machine has different voltage adjustments for each corresponding disease or ailment. The treatments are non-invasive, patient-friendly, and do not require a long time.

With the advent of artificial intelligence, many new changes in the treatment of cancer and other diseases will be introduced. This involves starting cancer treatment with the diet and the intestinal bacteria. Researchers now are finding that the diet, lifestyle, bacterial environment, metals, mineral deficiencies, fungus, parasites, and other causes of disease starts in the small intestine. They are finding the cause of the disease, type of intestinal bacteria, fungus, parasites, and other bad culprits.

This is the wonderful part. With the help of artificial intelligence and the new body, bacterial, and intestinal tests, they will find what kinds of bad bacteria, fungus, molds, parasites, and other conditions cause the toxic environment in the small intestine and body that causes cancer and other diseases. With these new tests and "AI," they will then be able to change the diet and bacterial flora, which is the basic cause of disease.

Regular physicians are not taught this new miracle that will come with artificial intelligence. They use mostly drugs, antibiotics, radiation, surgery, chemotherapy, chemo drugs, and lifestyle changes in their disease and cancer treatment. Please don't misunderstand me. Physicians do a tremendous job of wonderful treatments and help cure many diseases. We cannot get along without them. But many do not use preventive methods and diet to help prevent diseases before they develop into disease symptoms and full-blown diseases. Most of the problem lies in the diet, and the nasty guests in the small intestine, plus the toxins and inflammation which they produce.

This is where artificial intelligence will come into play. It will help in the testing, diagnosis, and defining the bacteria, metals, fungus, molds, candida, parasites minerals, vitamin deficiencies, and other causes of the problem. "AI," with many new tests, will find the cause, then doctors will prescribe the diet, probiotics, fermented foods, supplements, minerals, enzymes, vitamins, and other modalities needed to cure their disease or condition. In some cases, especially ulcerative colitis, they may use fecal transplants to treat or cure these ailments.

So how does a person start on this new paradigm of treatment? First, by taking many kinds of tests to find the cause of the symptom, disease, or condition. These tests will find the bad bacteria, fungus, molds, parasites, mineral deficiencies, vitamin deficiencies, environment, enzyme deficiencies, etc. which are causing the symptom, problem, disease, or condition.

Some of these tests, but not all are:

1. Stool tests

2. DNA and RNA tests.

3. Antibody tests.

4. Food intolerance tests.

5. Heavy metal tests.

6. Thyroid tests.

7. Hair analysis

8. VIOME test.

9. BRCA test for breast cancer

10. Reams (RBTI) test.

11. Blood and lipid tests.

12. Many other tests.

With the help of artificial intelligence, these tests will be interpreted and the results will show what the treatment needs to be. Many of these tests are revolutionary and are beginning to be available in most cities that have functional physicians and naturopaths.

Where do you go to get these treatments? If you are in a larger city, many functional medicine physicians, alternative cancer physicians, and naturopaths give many of these tests now. If you are in a smaller town, you may have to go to a larger city for now, until this type of treatment comes to your city or town. But it will come because it is the way disease can and will be treated in the future.

Don't be surprised if hemp CBD, CHD, and other cannabinoids start to be part of your symptom and cure treatment.

Be sure to keep up and read about artificial intelligence, medical tests, and cures now and in the future. There will be more future tests that will be very beneficial in finding diseases and conditions. The new medical treatments that are coming may save your life.

28

Proton Beam Radiation Therapy (PBT)

Proton beam radiation therapy is becoming more popular, especially for prostate, breast, and brain cancer. People who have had proton therapy and proton therapy physicians claim it is the safest and effective radiation treatment in the world. They claim it is much safer, with fewer side effects than regular radiation treatment.

About 20 PBT centers are now open in the United States. By 2021, it is estimated that worldwide, there will be about 100 centers.

Some of the benefits and non-benefits are 1. An advanced radiation treatment that reduces x-ray exposure to nearby tissues and organs. 2. It uses pencil-beam technology to attack cancer cells. 3. This highly precise radiation has fewer side effects than surgery or other radiation treatment. 4. A person can receive higher radiation doses with less exposure to healthy side tissue and organs. 5. It sends rapid pulses that are accurate within one millimeter to the exact spot of the tumor cells. 6. It reduces the scattered radiation dose. 7. It kills cancer cells by damaging the D.N.A. 8. Proton beams stop once they have delivered their energy to the target. 9. Anyone who can be treated with radiation therapy can be treated with PBT. 10. At present, PBT is currently used most in prostate, breast, and brain cancers. 11. Many patients who have had SURGERY for their prostate cancer become incontinent and many wish they had used proton beam therapy. 12. Some oncologists (not PBT physicians) say that there is not enough and complete enough data to show the effects and the result of treatment. 13. Proton therapy may be more expensive. It may not be covered by some insurances. 14. It does not guarantee that there will be no post-radiation side effects.

There is more and more information coming out about the benefits of proton therapy. It may be very worthwhile to check with one of the proton therapy clinics. You will be able to find them on the internet.

For more information, you can call the Loma Linda Cancer Center at 1 800 protons, or email them at www.protons.com.

29

References

1a Dr. Otto Warburg: Articles: "Cancer Research Papers" Amazon. Books: "The Prime Cause of Cancer," Amazon "The Metabolism of Tumors," Amazon

2a Dr. JoAnna Budwig: Book "Budwig Protocol," Amazon

3a 77 alternative Treatment doctors: Natural News, Feb. 15, 2016, Julie Wilson. According to snoops, this is unsubstantiated and has a lack of evidence.

4a Dr. Linus Pauling: Books: "General Chemistry," Find on eBay "Introduction to Quantum Mechanics," Linus Pauling and E. Bright Wilson, Jr. Find on eBay

5a Dr. Carey Reams: Book: "Choose Life or Death," Amazon

6a Dr. Jeffery Bradstreet: Several articles: "Therapeutic Role of Hematopoietic Stem Cells in Autism Spectrum Disorders-Related Inflammation," Siniscalco, D., Bradstreet, J.J., Antonucik N, "Frontiers in Immunology," 4.140 dols. 3389/fimmu (2013) 00140 PMC 3677147 PMID 23772227. "A Case-Control Study of Mercury Burden in Children with Autistic Spectrum Disorders," PDF Journal of American Physicians and Surgeons, Summer 2003, 8 (3) 76-79

7a Monsanto/Bayer Aspirin/Johnson lawsuit, Law firm; D. Miller and Associates. Class action lawsuit, Roundup 8a. 1. Nature of Medicine 24:1308, "Assessment of Glyphosate Induced Epigenetic Transgenerational Inheritance of Pathologies and Sperm Epimutations," "Generational Toxicology," Deeplko, Kubard, Eric E. Neilson, Stephanie E. King, Ingrid Saddler-Riggleman, Daniel Beck and Michael K Skinner. 2. "Scientific Reports," 2019, https://doi.org.10.1038/s41598-019-42860-0.

9a Bollinger, Tye: "The Truth about Cancer, What you Need to Know about Cancer History, Treatment and Prevention," Amazon, Kindle, Wikipedia

10a Dr. David Brownstein; Books: "Overcoming Thyroid Disorders, 3rd Addition,""Heal your Leaky Gut, the Cause of Many Chronic Diseases," Amazon

Section II

The Parent and Teacher Guide that Explain Nutrition Values in 54 Foods

I understand the complexity of keeping a person's body healthy and free of disease. The human body has millions of chemical reactions that occur in body cells, blood, organs, and the intestines.

In this section, each food, nutrient, or supplement group is rated according to the anionic or cationic energy they produce. This gives information which enables a person to buy and consume more high-electromagnetic foods that produce energy in the body cells, blood, organs and immune system. There are 54 groups of different foods, nutrients, and supplements, all rated at the top left as to the Electromagnetic Food (Card) Value, from 10 (highest) to 1 (lowest).

The upper left box contains the food's electromagnetic anionic or cationic value, depending on the energy produced, and the card number on the top right . The card numbers will be used for a Great Health and Nutrition Card Game that will be presented in the future.

Each food, nutrient and supplement group will have a written essay about the assets and liabilities of that group. At the bottom of the page (left) each food has a pH (energy strength) rating of acid, neutral, or alkaline. There is also a square on the bottom right showing the nutrition value of each food, nutrient and supplement group.

I am excited that you will be able to use the information on the following pages. You will be able to monitor the energy, pH and nutritional values. I hope that you will then be able to choose your food wisely.

Take care, my friend. Stay healthy and disease-free. An electromagnetic, ionic, neutral-pH diet on the following pages leads to a wonderful life of excitement, vitality, great energy, adventure, and longevity.

Table of Card Values

Card No.	Nutritional Value	Food, Nutrition or Supplement	pH Rating	Health Benefits
1.	15	Fresh ground flax, flaxseed oil mixed with kefir, and cottage cheese	100	Very high electromagnetic energy food, unravels sticky blood, stops inflammation and radical cell damage. Forms double bond carbon molecules. (Rx: 3-7 times/wk.)
2.	10	Fresh raw vegetables, fruit and vegetable juice	100	High alkaline and ionic properties, electromagnetic foods which contain minerals, vitamins, enzymes, amino acids and fiber. (Rx: 7 -11 daily)
3.	10	Raw, cold pressed norther seed oils, flaxseed, borage, Udo's choice, fish oil	100	Highly electromagnetic food helps control blood sugar, cholesterol inflammation and radical cell damage.
4.	10	Kefir, quark, plain yogurt, cottage cheese, fermented foods	100	Lactose intolerant, highly electromagnetic. Helps control blood sugar, cholesterol, inflammation and radical cell damage.
5.	10	Fresh organic apples, pears, peaches, berries, melons, and other fruits	100	Include in 7-11 diet with vegetables, antioxidant foods. Contain enzymes, and other polyphenols. Anti-inflammatory.
6.	10	Lemons, cucumbers, green drinks, vegetable juice and grapefruit	100	Creates alkaline enzymes, balanced pH. Produces calcium, Vitamin C and bicarbonate.
7.	10	Raw almonds, pecans, pumpkin seeds, walnuts, pistachios	100	Omega 3 oils, vitamins, minerals, antioxidants. Anti-inflammatory, polyunsaturated. (Rx: 3-4 of each daily)
8.	9	Pure water, distilled water, mineral water, (not bottled water)	98	Needed for all living organisms., Essential to keep optimum pH of blood and body cells. Essential for normal kidney and body functions. (Rx:3-4 glasses daily)
9.	9	Organic lemon juice, lime juice, kiwi, grapefruit juice	98	Contains vitamins, controls blood pressure, helps reduce kidney stones, breast and prostate cancer. Stimulates pancreas to produce alkaline enzymes.

10.	9	Extra virgin olive oil, coconut oil, palm oil	98	Reduces radical cell damage. Combats disease. Omega 3 oil. Keep in fridge. Coconut oil, palm oil, butter, best for cooking.
11.	9	Folic acid, B6, B12, D3	98	Folic acid, B6, B12 helps unravel sticky blood, (homocysteine). Helps prevent strokes, heart, attacks, phlebitis, HBP. (Rx: Folic acid, 800 mg, B6, 50 mg, B12, 500 mg, D3, 125 mg)
12.	9	Beans, peas, lentils, legumes	95	Best nutrition people can eat. Lowers blood, pressure, cholesterol, anti-inflammatory. Attacks free radicals, fiber. (Rx: eat often)
13.	8	Organic eggs	85	Great nutrition. Contains everything needed, in omega 3 oils, minerals, vitamins, amino, acids, enzymes, calcium, etc. (Rx: 3-8 per week)
14.	8	Garlic (allicin)	95	Great nutrition. Lowers blood pressure. Better than atenolol or warfarin, (BP pills). (Rx: 3-5 fresh cloves daily), decreases blood pressure.
15.	8	Raw apple juice, grape juice, red wine, other fresh raw juices	95	Contain many nutrients, polyphenols, vitamin C, minerals. Raises pH, Has vitamins, potassium. A very good source of nutrients and liquid.
16.	8	Wild game, deer, elk, moose, wild fish, salmon, sardines	95	Best source of protein. Little saturated fat, Contains omega 3 oils, minerals, calcium. Much better protein than pork and beef.
17.	8	Vegetable, steamed 3-8 minutes	95	Not as nutrient filled as raw veggies, but a great source of vitamins, enzymes, minerals, amino acids and other nutrients. Boil lightly.
18.	7	Organic avocados	95	Great ionic food. Helps stabilize blood sugar, lowers blood pressure, has omega 3 oils. Reduces cholesterol and triglycerides. Contains folic acid.
19.	7	Wobenzym – N Pancreatic enzymes	100	One of the great supplements. The benefits are enormous. Great for joints, intestinal bacteria, digestion and cancer prevention.

20.	7	Canned sardines, herring, free range eggs, legumes	95	Packed with vitamins, enzymes, minerals, amino acids, calcium, potassium, trace minerals, protein, and other nutrients. Suggest 4-8 eggs weekly. Does not raise cholesterol.
21.	7	Calcium Citrate, Calcium Orotate, Calcium Lactate, Calcium in food and cooked fish bones	95	Calcium is the king of minerals in your body. Raises pH, helps heart rhythm, bones, cartilage, brain. Regulates blood at 7.35 pH. Age over 45, I suggest calcium supplements.
22.	7	Cottage cheese, other white cheeses	90	Amazing fermented food. Mix with Kefir, flax seeds (crushed) & flaxseed oil; helps unravel sticky blood. Other cheeses good but not great. White cheeses are best.
23.	6	Vitamin C, Iodine, Vitamin D3	98	You need vitamin C daily. (see Linus Pauling) Vitamin D3 needed for brain function and development. 52 million Americans deficient in iodine.
24.	6	Magnesium, selenium, chromium	95	Calcium cannot be utilized W/O magnesium. Potassium needed. Prevents diabetes. Chromium, needed for long life. (Rx: All 3 daily)
25.	6	Xylitol, dark chocolate, coconut sweetener	85	Exit sugar. Use xylitol, coconut milk sweetener, dark chocolate. Has many minerals. nutrients
26.	6	poultry, farm raised	85	Much healthier if farm raised. Have no hormones, antibiotics, less omega 6 fat
27.	6	Turmeric, ginger	100	Turmeric: wonder supplement (curcumin). Over 20 healthy benefits. Slows inflammation, lowers blood pressure. Ginger has many good benefits. (Rx: 2 caps daily)
28.	15	Exercise, oxygen	100	Oxygen is very important for your health. The more oxygen, the more energy and health. Exercise 15+ minutes/day. Supplements: L-arginine, Ginkgo biloba, turmeric, periwinkle, all make NO2. Oxygen, Increases O2 to body cells. Check out hyperbaric Oxygen.

29.	5	Salsa, tomato sauce, tomatoes	65	Have lots of Vitamin C, lycopene. Recent studies have shown that tomatoes contain lectins which are toxic and inflame the gut wall.
30.	5	Pasteurized milk, milk	60	Pasteurized milk and products have very little value except for calcium. Raw milk is better. Has 44 antibodies plus other nutrients.
31.	5	Butter	80	10 times better for you than margarine. Butter contains butyrate, helps prevent colon cancer. One of best saturated fats for cooking.
32.	5	Canned vegetables	65	Good for you, but lose about 35%-40% of vitamins, enzymes, amino acids and other nutrients when cooked, depending on cooking time.
33.	4	Bananas, mangos, kiwi	65	Have lots of nutrients, minerals. Help control kidney function. Boost energy.
34.	4	Vegetables, boiled over 4 minutes	65	The longer veggies are cooked, the more nutrients are lost. Still very good for you. Keep eating them.
35.	4	Bread, breakfast cereal	40	One of oldest foods used on earth, All nutrition is in the husk. Flour turns to sugar in the intestines. Glycation. I suggest eating very sparingly.
36.	4	Coffee additives, Coffee creamers	45	Cream and almond milk are the best choices, Coffee creamers often have sugar and/or artificial sweeteners.
37.	4	Ice cream, shakes, sodas, whipped cream	20	Sweet and tasty. but contributes to HBP, diabetes, heart disease, arthritis, other diseases, cancer. Eat sparingly.
38.	3	Potatoes	25	Eaten throughout the world. They have some good traits, but raise glycemic index and have some lectins, Eat sparingly, but do not pass on them.
39.	3	Alcohol, hard drinks	10	Even though George Burns lived to 100 years, that doesn't mean they are good for you. They are a non-electromagnetic cationic (dead) food.

40.	3	Energy drinks, energy bars	25	Highly sweetened with sucrose, caffeine and preservatives. Non electromagnetic, cationic foods Can have excess caffeine. Some are good for energy. Choose wisely and sparingly.
41.	3	Hamburgers, deep fried chicken, fish etc.	15	No doubt, hamburgers, etc., are delicious, but they have (dead) cationic saturated oils, salt, cholesterol, and can cause sticky blood if eaten in excess.
42.	3	Red meat, pork	15	Can have good protein and iron, but saturated, (dead) cationic omega 6 oils. Otherwise, and if over 4 oz. will cause protease overload. Eat sparingly.
43.	2	Peanuts, cashews, macadamia nuts	5	Everyone loves nuts. Bad news: These nuts contain lectins. Lectins cause inflammation of the intestinal cell walls. Eat sparingly.
44.	2	All oils on the grocery shelf, except coconut, extra virgin olive oil, and butter	0	Pass up all oils on the grocery shelf, except coconut, palm, extra virgin olive oil, and butter. Cooked vegetable oils are saturated, non-electro- magnetic cationic (dead) oils. Bad for health.
45.	2	Processed foods, refined foods, microwaved foods	0	Produce acetic cationic ions. Non-electromagnetic. Acetic pH in body cells and organs. Nuked foods have no food value.
46.	2	Pies, cakes, Pudding, etc.	10	Very acidic, non-electromagnetic. Not good for your health. Very cationic, not healthy, eat sparingly.
47.	2	GMO soy, corn GMO products	0	Over 30,000 products should be banned, cause health. Very cationic. Not healthy. Eat sparingly. Government, FDA, Monsanto may be in collusion.
48.	−5	Cooking oils, salad dressing, lad, Crisco, mayonnaise, margarine	−5	These contain cationic (dead) non electromagnetic oils. Contain 30%-40% saturated omega 6 oils. Harmful to your health.

49.	1	Sugar, candy, sugar products	-5	Sugar causes candida and is cancer's best friend. Highly acetic. Non-electromagnetic, (dead) food. They cause high part of the disease process in humans.
50.	1	French fries, donuts, potato chips, other deep fried carbs	-5	95% cooked with acetic (dead) veggie oils. In excess cause HBP, heart disease, strokes, candida, parasites, leaky gut and other diseases
51.	1	Sausage, hotdogs	-5	These are tasty, but contain nitrates, omega 3 oils, preservatives plus cationic non electromagnetic omega 6 oils.
52.	1	Diet drinks, stevia, aspartame	-5	Nutritionists state; diet drinks # 1 enemy of health. Stevia, aspartame all acetic, non-electromagnetic (dead) foods.
53.	-5	Candida, cancer	-15	Feed your 25+ trillion intestinal bacteria non electro-magnetic acetic foods in excess and they will treat you with many candida, diseases and maybe cancer.
54.	+15	Intestinal bacteria	100	If you feed your 25+ trillion bacteria good electro-magnetic anionic food they will be very good to you, giving you an energetic, disease free, long life.

Seeds; Fresh Ground Flax and Chia, Plus Flaxseed Oil, Mixed with Quark and Cottage Cheese

In 1931, Dr. Otto Warburg discovered the cause of cancer. After Dr. Warburg's discovery. Dr. Linus Pauling discovered the alpha-helix carbon bond, which is the most energy-producing molecule in human food. The alpha-helix bond is responsible for many wonderful healing properties.

Following Dr. Pauling's work, Dr. Joanna Budwig discovered she could create a food mixture that used the alpha-helix bond molecules to help unravel sticky (homocysteine-laced) blood. Homocysteine (sticky blood) contributes to heart attacks, strokes, and cancer cell growth. Homocysteine in blood not only creates blood clots, but also creates a sticky blood which cannot carry oxygen to body cells. She found this contributes to cancer growth. She discovered that cancer loves low oxygen (an anaerobic environment), and thrives on foods that create an acetic body, glucose, and low oxygen.

She then discovered that the combination of these four foods: cottage cheese, flaxseed oil, quark, and crushed flaxseeds unraveled sticky blood and helped dissolve homocysteine. The result was an unraveling of the blood cells, so that more cancer-fighting oxygen would get to the body cells. This was a great discovery, for which she was nominated for the Nobel prize.

For her work on cancer, she was nominated for the Nobel prize six more times, but never got the prestigious award. These four mixed foods not only are needed to get rid of cancer, but are also critically important to prevent cancer, and to prevent blood clots, which cause heart attacks and strokes.

That is why I list them so highly, and believe they would help in everyone's diet if this combination was eaten two to four times a week for breakfast, (seven times per week with cancer). Two to four cut-up fruits may be added to improve the taste.

When flaxseeds (crushed in a coffee grinder) plus three tablespoons cottage cheese, two tablespoons flaxseed oil (mixed with electric mixer) are mixed with quark, it produces a very high-electromagnetic, anionic cell environment.

This mixture is water-soluble, and is easily absorbed into all blood and cell membranes. It helps in the program to cure cancer, prevent intestinal polyps, improve the immune system, create healthier intestinal bacteria, and prevent blood clots.

Dr. Budwig used this mixture to eradicate cancer in more than 2,500 patients, many of which were grade three and four cancer. Other practitioners had given up on them. Her cancer clinic in Germany still cures many cancer patients today, and can be found online.

To stay healthy, have a neutral ionic pH, increase good intestinal bacteria, help your immune system, plus prevent cancer and blood clots, it may be wise to consume the Budwig formula five to seven times each week. Keep all polyunsaturated oils in the refrigerator.

ELECTROMAGNETIC
GOOD DIET VOLTAGE
(pH) 6.2-6.8

NUTRITIONAL VALUE
[15]

[100%]
(100 – 50 Ionic)
(50 – 0 Cationic)

Seven to Eleven Fresh Raw Fruits, Veggies, Berries and Nuts Daily

Most biochemists agree that that man should be able to live on raw veggies, fruits, grains, seeds, legumes, nuts and water. With this diet, most people would be healthier, have a great immune system, very little disease, great intestinal bacteria, and live a long, healthy, good quality life.

But what went wrong with today's modern society? One hundred thousand refined and processed foods, sugar, candy, GMOs, cooked fats, alcohol, junk foods, etc., have diverted our perfect world into a world of obesity, candida, HBP, blood clots, diabetes, poor immune system and many diseases. In a perfect world, trees, plants and vegetables contain minerals, enzymes, vitamins, amino acids and fats. Eating these nutrients provides the basis for an electromagnetic, ionic, neutral-pH, healthy body system.

This is why I stress eating seven to eleven fresh fruits and vegetables each day. This may sound like fitting a square object into a round bowl, but it is not hard to get seven to eleven vegetables each day, if we make a salad once or twice each week, with a variety of fruits and vegetables. Add to that individual fruits and veggies for breakfast and snacks, and there you have it. Even if you have soups and other snacks during the day, it is not hard to get your seven to eleven veggies and fruits.

Many physicians, naturopaths, biochemists, and nutritionists are saying that 50 percent to 70 percent of your diet should contain fresh or lightly cooked vegetables, fruits, berries, melons, seeds, nuts and great polyunsaturated (omega-3) oils.

If every person in the United States would abide by these suggestions, our medical costs would be halved, to say the least.

What most people forget is that the grocery and food distributors have devised clever tricks to get you to stop and buy at the candy, fast food, refined food, and processed food counters. Educators have not devised criteria that help prevent disease states.

Electromagnetic ionic foods are the key to keeping you healthy and disease-free. Stopping at the produce counter will open the door to that healthy, disease-free life.

ELECTROMAGNETIC
GOOD DIET VOLTAGE
(pH) 6.2-6.8

NUTRITIONAL VALUE

[10]

[100]

(100 – 50 Ionic)

Raw Northern Seed Oils, Fish Oils, Borage, Flaxseed Oil

I cannot emphasize enough the importance of these raw, polyunsaturated (omega-3) seed and fish oils. They are essential for your diet, and should be found in your refrigerator and used every day. They are essential for your health in many ways. They are also essential to combat disease and keep your blood, body cells, and organs healthy and vital. These oils help form the alpha-helix bond carbon molecules that keep your cells healthy and full of energy. While helping to combat disease, they create ionic energy for your 25 trillion immune system bacteria. They help create the electromagnetic health essentials that run your body cells, blood, and organs. One or two teaspoons a day (especially flaxseed oil) mixed with cottage cheese, crushed flaxseeds, and quark (fermented goat or cow's milk) form an ionic mixture that is one of the best known foods to help prevent blood clots, inflammation, free-radical cell damage, disease, and cancer.

These polyunsaturated fats are not recommended for cooking. Cooking makes them prone to oxidation and free-radical changes in your body cells, organs, and blood. When cooking, one should use saturated oil because it does not produce free-radical changes. The best safe cooking oils are coconut oil, palm oil, and butter.

The polyunsaturated oils keep our intestinal bacteria happy and our immune system in great shape. Biochemists and nutritionists have found that one to one and one-half teaspoons of these polyunsaturated fats a day are essential for your body cells, heart, blood, organs, and immune system bacteria. They will combat blood sugar, inflammation, free-radical cell damage, toxicity, prostatitis, dementia, carpal tunnel, and many more health problems. They should be kept in the refrigerator and in dark bottles. Over time, if not kept cold, they will turn rancid and become dead omega-6 oils.

ELECTROMAGNETIC GOOD DIET VOLTAGE (pH) 6.2-6.8	NUTRITIONAL VALUE [10]	[100] (100 – 50 Ionic) (50-0 Cationic)

Organic Kefir, Cottage Cheese

When I think of kefir, I think of Kiefer Sutherland. But no, this kefir is a fermented milk drink, made from goat, cow or sheep's milk. The name kefir originated in the Caucasus mountains in Russia. Originally, it was started with quark curds, and put in canvas bags. It was then put in the doorway so it would get bumped when people went by to keep the mixture stirred and well mixed.

As a result of the fermentation, very little lactose was left in the kefir. Kefir is full of friendly probiotic bacteria, vitamins, calcium, and other minerals. French microbiologist Louis Pasteur is often mentioned for his work on fermentation, microbial growth and the production of microorganisms in probiotics, such as kimchi, yogurt, sauerkraut, champagne and wine. Fermentation enables foods to be easily predigested, so that when they are eaten, it requires less energy for them to be digested.

Kefir has other benefits. It helps control blood sugar, lowers cholesterol, and is a great probiotic, creating a healthier army of good bacteria in the intestines. Most people are not predisposed to eating these fermented foods. Believe me, to stay healthy and live a long life, they are very beneficial. They are a great source of natural organic probiotics, raise your body pH, provide several vitamins and minerals, plus help create energy and oxygen utilization.

Cottage cheese

Cottage cheese is made from milk with two different fat levels. There are two main types: large curd, with low acid, and small curd, with higher acid content.

Cottage cheese is high in protein, calcium, other minerals, and some vitamins. It is a very beneficial food when mixed with plain quark, crushed flaxseeds, and cold flaxseed oi. This mixture has a very high electromagnetic-energy ionic alkaline pH, which creates a alpha-helix bond molecule and helps unravel sticky blood.

ELECTROMAGNETIC GOOD DIET VOLTAGE (pH) 6.2-6.8

NUTRITIONAL VALUE [10]

[100]

(100 – 50 Ionic)

Raw Organic Cold Fresh Fruit, Berries and Melons

The old adage, "an apple a day keeps the doctor away" is surely true. A person's diet should include fruit, berries, and melons as part of the seven to eleven fruits and vegetables each day. I rate fruit, berries and melons, plus vegetables, as "electromagnetic superfoods." Most of them are also alkaline pH.

Some benefits of these great foods:

1. Most fruits, berries, and melons contain antioxidants, vitamins, enzymes, minerals, amino acids, and other nutrients, that combat intestinal inflammation and free-radical cell damage to the body cells.

2. The very high energy of these electromagnetic tasty morsels comes from polyphenols, flavonoids, vitamins, minerals, anthrocyanins, catachins and quercetins. In moderation, they also provide few calories.

3. Be sure to eat the skins. Much of the nutrition of these healthy electromagnetic foods is in the skin.

4. Strawberries are the only berries in the world that have their seeds on the outside of the berry.

5. These antioxidants have their origin in the ground. As explained in earlier chapters, the majority of the people in the US are acidic. This is an indication of a lack of eating these nutritious foods. The plant roots provide the many minerals, enzymes, amino acids, and other nutrients needed for acidic people to be pH-neutral.

6. Although most berries are edible, some berries are poisonous when not ripe. Others, such as nightshade and pokeweed, are poisonous when ripe.

7. Blueberries hold the top spot as a superfood. They are one of the most nutrient-dense foods you can eat. Besides being listed as having all the nutrients listed in number two, they are very high in vitamin C. I pick blueberries in the summer and freeze them in small packages for eating in the winter. These raw fresh fruits, berries and melons provide no plant fats.

8. Cucumbers and watermelons are two of the best foods for helping to raise an acid pH. They help raise the alkalinity.

9. These fruits, melons and berries are high in folate, vitamin B6, and B12. Varying your diet and adding supplements is usually necessary to get enough of these vitamins.

10. I recommend buying organic for all of these.

11. These foods are very healthful when dried, frozen, pickled, and better yet, as fresh as possible.

12. Please wash all of these foods before preparing them.

13. Cooking these fruits, berries and melons usually reduces the nutrition value 30 to 50 percent.

14. Fruits, berries and melons contain fructose. The advantage of fructose over sucrose is that it is released slowly.

The pancreas then has time to release insulin, and it is better for the pancreas and the body. The only harm may be in taking big portions

ELECTROMAGNETIC
GOOD DIET VOLTAGE
(pH) 6.8-7.0

NUTRITIONAL VALUE
[10]

[100]

(100 – 50 Ionic)

Lemons, Cucumbers, Broccoli, Watermelon, and Baking Soda

Baking soda in your diet? This may seem a little bit much, but many biochemists and nutritionists are saying that if your body is acidic (low pH) when you go to bed or get up in the morning, a little baking soda or lemon in a glass of water may help bring your low pH up to normal. Older people sometimes become very acidic, which is just the opposite of the neutral pH that a person should have when going to bed or getting up.

But you may not need to drink baking soda water to prevent acidity and keep an optimum neutral pH. Many fruits and vegetables contain potassium and sodium bicarbonate. Lemons, coffee, carrots, raisins, bananas, broccoli, asparagus, apples, grapes, cucumbers, and watermelons produce bicarbonate and potassium, which help raise the alkalinity (pH) of your blood and body cells. These foods also help reduce lactic acid, which contributes to fatigue, inflammation and free-radical damage to your body cells.

Why do we think that lemon, cucumbers, broccoli and watermelon are so important? They are the highest alkaline helpers, and they raise your pH when your body may be anxious to become acidic. Most diseases, HBP, diabetes, heart and stroke problems, plus cancer, all prosper in an acid environment. More importantly, the intestinal bacteria are compromised in an acid environment, and good bacteria cannot multiply for your healthy digestion and good immune system. Your digestive bacteria ratio needs to be 80 percent good to 20 percent bad, in order to provide excellent digestion of food and keep a healthy immune system.

Acidity will lower the ratio of good to bad bacteria in your intestines, creating a disease and Candida-friendly environment. If your body is acetic at night (low pH) a great help is to put 2 tablespoons of pure lemon juice or tablespoon of soda in a cup of water and drink it. This is a great habit for older people who tend to get more acetic when eating the average American diet. Low acetic people should make soda, lemons, cucumbers, broccoli, and watermelon frequent visitors to your refrigerator, table and diet.

1. Cucumbers and watermelons are two of the best foods for helping to raise the alkalinity when you have an acid pH.

2. These fruits and melons are high in folate, vitamin B6, and B12. Varying your diet with these vitamins, plus adding supplements, may be wise for older people.

3. I recommend buying all these foods organic.

4. These foods are very healthful when dried, frozen, pickled and better yet, as fresh as possible.

5. Please wash all of these fruits, berries and melons before preparing them.

6. Cooking these fruits, berries and melons usually reduces the nutrition value 30 percent to 50 percent.

7. Fruits, berries and melons contain fructose. The advantage of fructose over sucrose is that it is released in your intestines slowly. The pancreas has time to release insulin. that is better for the pancreas and the body. The only harm may be in taking very large portions.

ELECTROMAGNETIC
GOOD DIET VOLTAGE
(PH) 6.8-7.0

NUTRITIONAL VALUE
[10]

[100]

(100 – 50 Ionic)

Raw Almonds, Pecans, Walnuts, Macadamia Nuts, and Pistachios

Some of the simplest foods are the greatest for your health. This really is true with nuts. It would be good to eat some of these great superfoods every day. These nuts are some of the most essential foods you can eat. I suggest that you eat two to three of these raw nuts every day. I have eaten two to three of these nuts every day for many years, and can only say they have provided many nutrients and great omega-3 fats. Eating them raw every day provides a great good-bacterial boost, and helps every cell in your body. You can keep them in the fridge or freezer. Although they all have a lot of nutrients, they vary from nut to nut. They are high in monounsaturated omega-3 fats, calcium, manganese, copper, omega-7 palmitoleic acid, thiamine, iron, vitamin E, folate, protein, vitamin E, and many lesser nutrients. Wow. They really are super.

The many things they do:

1. Reduce heart attacks, strokes, and blood clots in the veins.

2. Lower bad cholesterol and protect artery walls from damage.

3. Help build strong bones and teeth.

4. Lower the risk of diabetes.

5. Help provide good brain function.

6. Great digestive helpers that nourish good bacteria.

7. Lowers blood pressure.

8. Have oleic acid, which helps prevent breast and prostate cancer.

9. Powerful antioxidants which battle intestinal inflammation and leaky gut.

10. These nuts contain L-arginine, which produces nitric acid, and allows the blood to carry more oxygen to the body cells and organs.

Other good nuts are pine nuts, brazilnuts, and hazelnuts. Peanuts and cashews contain lectins and aflatoxins, and do not have as much nutrition as other nuts.

ELECTROMAGNETIC
GOOD DIET VOLTAGE
(pH) 6.2-6.8

NUTRITIONAL VALUE
[10]

[100]

(100 – 50 Ionic)

Water

A universal solvent is one that affects all people and remarkably, the entire earth. It is applicable to all purposes, conditions, and situations. That, my friends, is the definition of water.

We cannot live without water, and it is wise to drink three to three liters of water or water equivalent every day. A chronic deficiency of water may result in chronic acidity, and also in possible damage to the kidneys and kidney function.

More importantly, the pH of water (7.4) is the ideal pH of the blood and body cells. It is needed for keeping a neutral body pH plus keeping an ideal urine and body pH at 6.2 to 6.8.

A lack of water in your body may influence your pH by lowering the normal saliva and urine pH, causing more acidity, inflammation, and free-radical cell damage. The inflammation and free-radical cell damage promote disease.

The best source of water for humans is distilled water. If you are drinking water from a city source, it may have harmful impurities, including mercury, fluorine, chlorine, lead, aluminum, and sometimes, unhealthy bacteria. It may be wise to check with the city water officials to see how and when they check the water for impurities. They should show you the tests. If you are drinking water from a well, it is wise to get the water tested for impurities every six or eight months. Many nutritionists and naturopaths suggest that a person drink distilled water, because it has no impurities, toxins, or metals. Drinking water in plastic bottles or containers may be good, but the bisphenol in the plastic contains estrogen. Over time, drinking bottled water could lead to excess exposure to estrogen, and estrogen in excess has been known to trigger prostate and breast cancer.

A few of the great things that water does for your body:

1. It helps get rid of body toxins.

2. Helps increase energy in the body.

3. Helps regulate body temperature.

4. Helps regulate body pH.

5. Helps in weight loss.

6. Helps in production of good intestinal bacteria.

7. Helps decrease urinary tract infections.

ELECTROMAGNETIC GOOD DIET VOLTAGE (pH) 6.8-7.4

NUTRITIONAL VALUE [9]

[100]

(100 – 50 Ionic)

Fresh Organic Citrus Juices, Apple Juice, and Organic Cider Vinegar

Just about everyone knows that raw, fresh citrus fruits contain vitamin C and help prevent scurvy. However, they do a lot more for your health. What many people may not know is that these fruits can help reduce breast and stomach cancer, lower blood pressure, and reduce some kidney stones. Vitamin C, which has multiple cellular uses, is known for its Krebs cycle (citric acid cycle). The Krebs cycle is a series of chemical reactions where the end result is the manufacture and storage of energy. The end product, adenosine triphosphate (ATP) is the energy product needed for our bodies to operate. The Krebs cycle also manufactures precursors to certain amino acids, which participate in cellular metabolism and energy. Processed juices do not hack it.

There are two wonderful actions of raw, fresh citrus fruits, organic apple cider vinegar, and pure, raw citrus juices. One is the production of channel blockers, helpful in reducing high blood pressure. Actually, citrus fruits, garlic, and magnesium all help as channel blockers, maybe as well as any medications. Another wonderful action of citrus fruits and organic apple cider vinegar is the stimulation of the pancreas to produce alkaline enzymes. These are a great help in raising the body, blood, and cellular pH, needed for people to lower an acidic, non-electromagnetic pH. Organic apple cider vinegar is a fermented juice that contains vitamin C, B6, B12, biotin, folate, and niacin (wow!). It also contains many minerals: sodium, phosphate, magnesium, calcium, iron, and zinc. In addition, it also lowers high blood pressure and blood sugar levels, helps in weight loss, and reduces acne. It is good for toxin elimination and for arthritis.

If you do not have these miracle juices in your refrigerator, you are missing the Goliaths of the juice world!

Coconut Oil, Palm Oil, and Butter

If you want to use an oil that seems to be very good, especially for cooking, then coconut oil is one of the best. Coconut oil is a saturated oil. However, it is a very stable oil for cooking, and does not show any molecular change when heated. It is by far a better oil than any monounsaturated or polyunsaturated oil for that purpose. Many biochemists and nutritionists recommend coconut oil for cooking. Virgin, cold-pressed, unrefined coconut oil in small amounts also provides some good benefits when consumed. It is said to be helpful to balance the polyunsaturated oils in combating inflammation and free-radical cell damage.

There are two other great oils for cooking. They are palm oil and butter. Cooking oils need to stay stable and undergo few molecular changes when heated. Both palm oil and butter fit that category.

Polyunsaturated and monounsaturated oils are very unstable when used for cooking. Also, all oils on the grocery shelf (except extra virgin olive oil) are unstable, non-electromagnetic, dead oils, and should not be used for cooking.

Heating these oils creates trans and megatrans fats, which cause inflammation and free-radical damage to your body cells. It is wise to keep all eating and cooking oils in the refrigerator

ELECTROMAGNETIC
GOOD DIET VOLTAGE
(pH) 6.9-7.2

NUTRITIONAL VALUE
[9]

[98]

(100 – 50 Ionic)

[9]   **Electromagnetic Food**   **Card**
Nutrition   **#11**
Value

Folate, Vitamin B6, and B12, the Unraveling Vitamins

Folate is found in leafy green vegetables and liver. It is essential in treating anemia and neural tube maladies in children. The real important function of folate (B9), B6, and B12 is in the reduction of cardiovascular disease, including strokes, blood clots, and heart attacks. There is a substance in the blood that is a clotting factor in heart disease. It is called homocysteine. Folate, B6, and B12 help to control homocysteine and unravel the blood, helping to reduce blood clots. An important factor is that these three supplements, while unraveling the blood, enable the blood to carry more oxygen to the body cells. This is a big factor, as candida fungus helps in the formation of sticky blood and low body cell oxygen. In recent research, the results of a poor diet, candida manifestation, and low body oxygen have been shown to be a factor in the development of cancer. Folate, B6, and B12 are so important that it may be wise to consider taking these supplements every day.

Another very important function of folate is to help create DNA and RNA, both of which are very essential in the metabolism of amino acids. B6 and folate are also essential nutrients that are coenzymes in more than 100 enzyme reactions in the body. They are very important in hemoglobin synthesis and function, as well as in neurotransmitter function.

B6 is found in raw animal and plant food. Cooking, heating, and processing of B6 results in the lost of most of the B6. Vitamin B12 (cobalamin) is one of the most essential vitamins.

Along with vitamin D3, they have a key role in the development and function of the brain and nervous system. B12 is essential for the metabolism of every cell in the body. It helps in the synthesis of DNA, folate, and amino acids. Food sources are shellfish, organ meats and liver.

Suggested dosages: Folate: 800 mg/day; B6, 50 mg/day, and B12, 50 mg/day.

Beans, Peas, Lentils and Other Legumes

Many Americans do not eat enough legumes. They eat a lot of refined foods that have little or no food value, and are loaded with preservatives, sucrose, corn syrup, and other non-electromagnetic foods.

Legumes are not only a great healthy electromagnetic food, but the best nutrition that anyone could eat, three to four times during the week. Red beans, navy beans, black-eyed peas, dried peas, black beans, lima beans, lentils, other legumes, and even soy (as long as it is organic and non-GMO), are not only a great source of protein and fiber, but are full of vitamins, and a great alkaline food that can help create a pH-neutral body.

In some countries where people eat large quantities of legumes, they live to be very old, and attribute their long lives to these tasty morsels. One of the reasons legumes are very good is that they help reduce inflammation and free-radical damage to the body cells. This is a great benefit in the reduction of disease. Most people who eat a lot of beans, peas, lentils, and other legumes also have lower levels of cholesterol, lower blood pressure, and a lower glycemic index. They have less arthritis and diabetes, especially if they are not a sugar addict, and do not eat a lot of carbohydrates and refined foods. Legumes have many great benefits. They have a lot of wonderful fiber, protein, organic micronutrients, and phytonutrients.

Even soy, if it is not a GMO derivative, has lots of benefits, including phyto- estrogens, which, in some studies, reduce breast and prostate cancer. You have to be careful with soy, as 90 percent of all soy is now a GMO food, so watch for organic soy when you buy. One real disadvantage is that the government and the FDA do not make the food companies put GMO labels on soy and corn products. One thing to remember: vegetable diets usually lack vitamin B12. Vegetarians are urged to take B6, B12, and folate as supplements to their daily diet. I hope you are not waiting to start putting beans, peas, and other legumes in your diet.

They are a great electromagnetic energy food. They really are the miracle fruit.

ELECTROMAGNETIC
GOOD DIET VOLTAGE
(pH) 6.8-7.2

NUTRITIONAL VALUE
[9]

[98]

(100 – 50 Ionic)

Organic and Farm-Raised Chickens and Eggs

There is a lot of difference between farm-raised animals and birds versus caged (penned) ones. Penned animals and birds are fed hormones and antibiotics, since they live in such close quarters. Also, the muscle tissue has more omega-6 fats. Farm-raised chickens and eggs are far more nutritious than pen-raised. Farm-raised eggs can be one of the healthiest parts of your diet. The old nutrition books that say eggs are responsible for high cholesterol seem to be out of date.

Researchers have found that omega-6 fats, dead, cooked vegetable oils, excessive red meats, sugar products, and refined carbohydrates are more responsible for high cholesterol levels, triglycerides, and high blood pressure. Since eggs have all the nutrients, minerals, vitamins, enzymes, calcium, proteins, etc., to produce a chicken, they surely are a very nutritious food, containing almost all of the proteins and fats that are good for your health. Eggs contain almost everything to help you acquire good nutrition.

Very important, however, is that they are much more healthful if raw, lightly boiled or lightly fried. Cooking destroys many essential vitamins, enzymes, amino acids, essential oils, and other nutrients. Raw eggs or lightly cooked eggs contain a substance called APO 1, 2, and 3. Those substances have an affinity for mercury and help the body excrete mercury.

Raw or lightly cooked, boiled, or poached eggs also seem to retain more polyunsaturated fats, vitamin A, and vitamin C, plus many other good nutrients. Excessive cooking, prolonged hard boiling, or eggs fried too long are not as nutritious as raw, lightly boiled, or lightly fried. Raw eggs can be mixed in a mixture and added to many other mixed foods. Farm-raised organic chickens are also far better for you than when pen-raised. Farm-raised chickens and eggs can be a great addition to your diet.

ELECTROMAGNETIC
GOOD DIET VOLTAGE
(pH) 6.2-6.8

NUTRITIONAL VALUE
[8]

[85]

(100 – 50 Ionic)

Garlic (Allicin)

I hope you do not get a bitter taste in your mouth about garlic. The reason is that I cannot begin to state the wonderful benefits that garlic provides for your body and health. It should be labeled electromagnetically a 15. Garlic contains a sulfur compound called allicin. Allicin is an antifungal. However, the allicin is imprisoned in the garlic until it is squeezed in a garlic squeezer or chopped fine with a vegetable chopper. This activates the garlic so the allicin can be released and assimilated in the intestines, body and the body cells.

The incredible list of garlic benefits should warrant serious and careful consideration, for consuming two to four raw cloves of garlic every day in salad, vegetables, or other foods.

1. It is an antifungal plus antibacterial food, and helps eradicate bad bacteria and candida in your intestines. candida fungus is the driver of poor health and cancer. Garlic is a superfood, which is at least as good or more effective than most fungicides.

2. Garlic stabilizes blood sugar, reduces inflammation and slows free radical cell damage in the body cells. It improves insulin sensitivity, while keeping the blood pressure down. This helps in controlling heart and blood vessel disease.

3. It helps prevent blood clots, strokes and heart attacks. Two to four raw crushed cloves (not cooked) a day in salad, or mixed food work as good as atenolol or warfarin in protecting the blood vessels, heart and circulation. Most blood pressure medications have side effects, which are absent with garlic. Garlic also helps in treating type II diabetes and liver damage,

4. It helps support the alveoli in the lungs and prevents congestion.

5. It supports a healthy pancreas and insulin production.

6. If you cannot take raw fresh garlic in food, three capsules of garlic supplements every day would be sufficient to make up the difference. I suggest the Garlic Plex from Daily Manufacturing as a very effective supplement.

Conclusion: Garlic is the Superman and Wonder Woman of all foods. Eating crushed or chopped garlic every day is like taking an army of supplements, all in two to four garlic cloves.

ELECTROMAGNETIC
GOOD DIET VOLTAGE
(pH) 6.8-7.2

NUTRITIONAL VALUE
[8]

[100]

(100 – 50 Ionic)

[8]   **Electromagnetic Food**   **Card**
Nutrition   **#15**
Value

Grapes, Red and White Wine, Fresh Organic Apple Cider

Wines contain many nutrients, including polyphenols that seem to be very beneficial to the residents of Italy, Greece, France, the United States, and many other countries. White wines are preferred by many people, especially in the U.S. They have been recommended for many types of meals depending on the host or restaurant. White wines have the same alcohol content as red wines but have a lesser amount of good nutrients. Red, white wines, and champagne are fermented. Champagne is, in fact doubly fermented. It is easier for your body to digest fermented foods and liquids. However, please do not use this as a reason for overindulgence. Red wines and red champagne lack the nutrients and minerals of raw grapes since the majority of nutrients and minerals are in the skin of the grape. The skin produces the color of the grape and contains the yeast responsible for the fermentation. In red grapes, the skin also contains anthocyanins, polyphenols, tannins, minerals, and vitamin C. Also present in grapes is vitamin B1, which is necessary for the action of the yeast in the fermentation. Red wine is said to be helpful in small or moderate amounts with cardiovascular benefits and the reduction of low-density lipids (LDL). Wine is not nearly as helpful nutritionally, as organic grapes.

Organic Apple Cider

An apple a day keeps the doctor away, or so they say. Raw, fresh, organic apple juice (not concentrated) has many benefits. It contains fiber, acetic acid, minerals, vitamin C, polyphenols, and quercetin. It helps raise the body pH, helps the good bacteria in your intestines become more prolific, more productive, and multiply faster. It also helps in the prevention of cancer and other diseases, plus reduces obesity.

ELECTROMAGNETIC
GOOD DIET VOLTAGE
(pH) 6.8-7.2

NUTRITIONAL VALUE
[8]

[95]

(100 – 50 Ionic)

Wild Game, Birds, Fish, Salmon, Trout

Prehistoric man and indigenous tribes made wild game birds, meat, and fish a staple in their diet. Some anthropology books even state that they think the reason man's brain and intelligence evolved ahead of all other animals was that they ate a diet of more protein.

The first white men that came up the Columbia river in the north-western US saw millions of salmon spawning. They said you could smell the dead fish a quarter mile away from the river. They also saw racks and racks of salmon and wild meat, hanging on the racks to dry for the Indians' winter staples.

Wild birds, game and fish are constantly on the move. This enables the muscle to be dense, with very little fat. That is a great attribute, since excessive interstitial fat in wild meat can have a better ratio of omega-6 to omega-3 fat.

Wild game, birds, and fish contain very little omega-6 fat (6 to 10 percent) while pen-raised beef, pork, and chicken can have from 30 to 50 percent omega-6 fat. The optimum human ratio for omega-6 to omega-3 should be between 2 to 1 and 3 to 1 in the body. Excessive omega-6 fat consumption in humans can result in intestinal inflammation and oxidation of body cells, excessive candida fungus, high blood pressure, autoimmune diseases, lowering of the immune system, and many other health problems.

Compared to pen-raised beef and pork, wild game wins the good fat and oil contest. It provides much better omega-3 oils, plus more protein and less omega-6 saturated fats. I judge wild game, birds and fish way above their domestic pen-raised cousins. It wouldn't hurt to have wild (not pen-raised) fish, wild birds, and chicken 2-4 times a week.

ELECTROMAGNETIC
GOOD DIET VOLTAGE
(pH) 6.2-6.8

NUTRITIONAL VALUE
[15]

[96]

(100 – 50 Ionic)

Vegetables, Fruit, Steamed or Boiled

Steaming foods is one of the healthiest cooking methods, yet most people boil their vegetables and fruit rather than steaming them. Steaming is an easy, yet relatively quick way to be rewarded with wonderful nutrient-filled food. It is said that steamed vegetables will retain a few more nutrients over boiling. Vegetables and fruit steamed or boiled lose some of the vitamins, amino acids, and enzymes. It is estimated that the loss is about 30 percent to 40 percent of the electromagnetic and nutrient content, if not overboiled. Still, vegetables steamed or boiled are a great way for older citizens and people with a poor chewing ability to get some good nutrition. It takes more cooking time for some vegetables to cook before they are palatable. Below are some of the approximate cooking times for some of the different vegetables. However, space constraints do not allow the cooking times for all vegetables and fruit.

It is important to remember that overcooking and/or long cooking times will destroy more and more of the vitamins, enzymes, amino acids, and other nutrients, so it is important to cook the vegetables and fruit the minimum palatable time to get the best nutrients from the food.

1. Asparagus, 7 to 12 minutes

2. Cauliflower, 6 to 9 minutes

3. Broccoli, 6 to 9 minutes

4. Carrots, 12 to 16 minutes

5. Beets, 14 to 16 minutes

6. Corn, 6 to 9 minutes

7. Green beans, 7 to 10 minutes

8. Cabbage (cut), 7 to 10 minutes

9. Beet greens, 6 to 10 minutes

10. Brussels sprouts, 8 to 10 minutes

[7]   **Electromagnetic Food**   **Card**
Nutrition   **#18**
Value

Organic Avocados

Don't overlook avocados. They are one of the most important foods you could eat. As one of the best sources of polyunsaturated electromagnetic oils, they contain palmitic, linoleic, and oleic acid, which help regulate blood sugar. There are many wonderful reasons you should have avocados on your plate, three to five times weekly. Here are some of the great things they do:

1. Stabilize blood sugar and blood pressure

2. Reduce LDL cholesterol and triglycerides.

3. Plays a major role in cancer prevention

4. It contains amazing polyunsaturated oils and helps reduce blood sugar.

5. Helps in weight loss.

6. They contain folic acid (folate), helping make new healthy body cells, plus reduces sticky (homocysteine) blood.

7. The perfect baby food.

8. Has lots of carotenoids, lutein, and antioxidants

9. Helps produce healthy skin and hair

10. Helps smooth wrinkles.

11. Contain phytosterols such as lutein and Ianthinine.

12. Even the pit, when broken down in a blender, contains phenolic compounds used to treat inflammation and free radical oxidation in body cells, plus helps diabetes and high blood pressure. Even better, avocados showed a decrease in serum cholesterol levels, a 22 percent decrease in total LDL plus an eleven percent increase in HDL. If you do not have avocados

in your fridge or pantry now, it may be wise to head to the grocery store. Make sure they are ripe but not overripe

ELECTROMAGNETIC
GOOD DIET VOLTAGE
(pH) 6.2-6.8

NUTRITIONAL VALUE

[7]

[95]

(100 – 50 Ionic)

155

Wobenzym-N and Pancreatic Enzymes

If you want to provide yourself and your family with the best preventive cancer supplement on the market, you might give your family wobenzym-N tablets. The active ingredients of this wonderful supplement are several enzymes, trypsin, pancreatin, chymotrypsin, papain, bromelain, and rutin. All of these pancreatic enzymes help your poor overworked pancreas digest your foods.

One of the extremely important preventive and alternative cancer treatments, wobenzym-N, and other pancreatic enzymes (including solozyme and pepsin) has had great success in the treatment and elimination of cancer cells. Cancer cells use all of the body's enzymes to metabolize the protein needed for the cancer cell production plus enzymes to digest the protein they steal from body muscles. A big part of preventive cancer and cancer treatment is treating the deficiency of pancreatic enzymes. Without supplemental enzymes, there are not enough pancreatic enzymes for the digesting of a person's food when they have cancer. Cancer cells love sugar, protein, and low oxygen. They are selfish cancer and blood scavengers. Excess pancreatic enzymes are also needed to prevent and/or stop cancer cell hits. With cancer, 12 to 18 enzymes a day are suggested between meals. If you have cancer, you can get solozymes from 817 458 9241 or www.collegehealthstores.com Wobenzym-N enzymes can be found on the internet.

Enzymes are biological catalysts that play a critical role in digesting food. 15,000 enzymes and 30 million chemical reactions take place every time you eat food. Enzymes are involved in most of our metabolic processes. Wobenzym-N and its concentrated enzymes also help balance a natural inflammation process, plus helps in joint relief and arthritis. It helps control swelling and pain.

It may be wise to consider wobenzym-N as a very valuable supplement that should be taken every day. My wife and I each take three tabs daily.

ELECTROMAGNETIC
GOOD DIET VOLTAGE
(pH) 6.2-6.8

NUTRITIONAL VALUE
[15]

[100]

(100 – 50 Ionic)

Canned or Dried Sardines, Herring, Salmon, and other Fish

Don't forget to buy some canned sardines, salmon, or herring on your next trip to the grocery store. It is best to have them cooked in water. They are packed with electromagnetic goodies, including calcium, vitamins, minerals, enzymes, amino acids, and omega 3 oils. One canned sardine, herring, or four 0unces of canned salmon gives you 500 milligrams of calcium, much protein, daily percentage of vitamin B12, phosphorus, potassium, trace minerals, and other nutrients.

When the first two white men from the Hudson's Bay Company canoed their way more than 200 miles up the Columbia River around 1812, they encountered 18 Indian tribes living along the river. Many of the Indians had never seen a white man, and most tribes were very friendly. Many tribes would even butcher a dog and have a great feast, welcoming the new white men. However, there were two very unfriendly tribes. The friendly tribe members would warn the traders ahead of time, so they could forage their canoe and supplies around the unfriendly tribes. It would take a lot of time.

The Hudson's Bay traders found that thousands of salmon were spawning all along the banks of the Columbia. So many had died after spawning that the traders could smell the dead salmon a quarter of a mile away. All of the Indian tribes netted and speared hundreds of salmon. They dried them on rows of long poles and saved most of them for the coming winter.

The salmon contained great omega 3 oils, calcium, vitamins, minerals, enzymes, and amino acids, giving the tribes protein and sustenance for the winter. The Indian tribes knew what great electromagnetic energy foods these fish were. The same applies to sardines, herring, and other canned fish. They are a great source of omega 3 oils and other nutrients. They are very good for you frozen or fresh.

ELECTROMAGNETIC
GOOD DIET VOLTAGE
(pH) 6.2-6.8

NUTRITIONAL VALUE
[7]

[95]

(100 – 50 Ionic)

Calcium, One of the Most Important Minerals in the Body

Calcium is needed in several ways in the body. It is not only the foundation of our structure, but is an important electrolyte that controls the rhythm of our heart and is needed in all muscles, bone formation, neurotransmission in body movements, pancreatic function, brain function, digestion, bone formation, and density, plus much, much more.

One very important problem is the relationship to the acidity of your body (low pH of urine and saliva below 6.2). Chronic cationic body acidity causes a very big calcium problem, and it needs to be explained what happens when there are an uneven bite and calcium deficiency along with a cationic (acidic) body. Excess sugar, carbohydrates, and red meat may expedite this problem.

Electrolyte conduction controls the rhythm of your heart. It is very essential and critical for the blood pH to maintain a pH reading of 7.4. When a person has a very acidic body (urine and saliva pH less than 6.2), the blood pH can get lower than 7.4. When that happens, since the heart has to maintain a constant 7.4 pH and rhythm, the blood sends out signals to obtain more calcium in the blood, to raise the pH. This is where it gets very dicey. Where does the extra calcium come from? It has to come from areas of infection and/or trauma (using osteoclasts) somewhere in the body. Where does that infection and/or trauma occur in an acidic body? It occurs between the teeth (gum infections, grinding, trauma) or in the cartilages, between the cervical vertebrae. People with temporal mandibular dysfunction have trauma because their posture changes, not only causing neck muscle strain but headaches and neckaches. With a low acidic pH, the neck trauma releases tiny osteoclasts (blood bone destroyers) that break down the periodontal bone and cervical cartilages. The calcium is released into the blood to raise the blood (heart rhythm) pH to 7.4. The calcium deficiency may cause a herniation or perforation of the vertebral cartilages. Eventually, if the calcium loss and bite are not corrected, it will cause the cervical vertebral meniscus to require surgery to get rid of the pain symptoms (not the cause). However, the real cause is the bad dental bite, acidity, calcium deficiency, plus temporal mandibular dysfunction, and dysfunctional posture.

Between the teeth and cervical vertebral area, this osteoclastic release of cartilage/bone calcium can also occur in the lower lumbar area when a person has scoliosis or accident in the lower back.

People need to realize that an acidic body plus low serum calcium is a serious problem. This condition also exists in older people when they get osteoporosis. People start to lose calcium after the age of 45. After age 45 it is important to know that added calcium may be necessary to replace the calcium that is lost. It is very important not to let your calcium reserve get too low. Osteoporosis is very common in older people, especially if their saliva and urine pH gets below 6.2 and the person eats a high acetic diet, especially with excess sugars, carbohydrates, and red meats. Weak bones can cause accidents.

It is also very important to know that magnesium, potassium, zinc, and vitamin D3 are calcium helpers and very essential for older people. I suggest dosages of calcium, 400 to 600 mg, magnesium, 100 to 400 mg, and D3, 400 to 800 IU. Some types of calcium do not assimilate very well in the body. Oyster shell calcium and Tums may be alkaline but are not the best sources of calcium. Since there are so many forms of calcium, it may be wise to have a certified nutritionist or health professional help find the best-suited calcium for you to maintain a neutral pH. If that is not possible, there is much useful neutral calcium. Some of those are calcium aspartate, calcium citrate, calcium gluconate, calcium phosphate, and calcium orotate. A very good source of calcium is cottage cheese, canned sardines, herring, and salmon. The bones in most canned fish contain supplemental calcium.

A person should not take calcium supplements in excess. That may cause hypercalcemia and digestive problems.

ELECTROMAGNETIC
GOOD DIET VOLTAGE
(pH) 6.2-6.8

NUTRITIONAL VALUE
[7]

[95]

(100 – 50 Ionic)

Low Fat Cottage Cheese, Other Cheeses

The first known use of cottage cheese dates back to 1831. Since cottage cheese is a fermented food, it is an amazing nutrient. A four-ounce serving contains two to four percent milk fat, 120 calories, five grams of saturated fat, three grams of carbohydrates, twelve grams protein, seventy grams calcium, 500 mg. sodium, twenty mg. cholesterol, and trace amounts of potassium and phosphorous. This makes cottage cheese a very nutritious food.

One great advantage of low-fat cottage cheese is that it can be mixed with kefir, flaxseed oil, and/or ground flaxseeds to make a very high double bond helix carbon molecule. It is highly electromagnetic. This mixture thins sticky (homocysteine) blood. Many German physicians use this mixture for treating heart disease and cancer. It should be high on your daily menu.

Other Cheeses

Cheese is made from cows and other mammals including goats, camels, sheep, reindeer, and yaks. The origin of cheese dates back more than 6,000 years. There is a very wide variety of cheeses available for your diet. Most cheeses have some very good nutrients including one-third of a person's daily requirement of calcium, 10 percent to 14 percent protein, calcium, phosphorus, and saturated fat. Different studies have had conflicting results as to the nutrient and digestive value of cheeses. Some say that most cheeses increase and help contribute to saturated fats and LDL cholesterol. Later studies state that these fermented cheeses lower LDL.

Mozzarella cheese is the most popular cheese in the United States. This is probably due to the large amounts of pizzas consumed by the populace. Some of the other popular cheeses are parmesan, ricotta, feta, provolone, Monterey Jack, brie, Swiss, and gruyere. It is good for pregnant women to go real slow on cheese. I suggest: enjoy cheese but go slow on cheeses and pizzas.

ELECTROMAGNETIC GOOD DIET VOLTAGE (pH) 6.2-6.8

NUTRITIONAL VALUE [7]

[90]

(100 – 50 Ionic)

Vitamin C, Vitamin D3, and Iodine

I don't want to overlook the importance of vitamin C. My chapter on Linus Pauling tells the story of why Vitamin C is so helpful in a person's quest for health and longevity. It is also covered in the five foods a person should get. It is a very important supplement: Preventive recommendation, 2000 mg per day

Vitamin D3

Vitamin D is known as the 'sunshine vitamin." It is produced in your skin in response to the ultraviolet rays of the sun. However, many people do not get much sunshine, and in those cases, supplemental vitamin D3 may be needed. You can also get vitamin D3 from some foods, but it is wise to rely on supplements if you have not been exposed to much sunlight.

Vitamin D3 is essential for brain development and is direly needed for pregnant women and young infants. It has been found recently that a hormone, nagalase, has been added to some infant vaccination material. Unfortunately, one of the physicians who discovered this problem mysteriously died.

Nagalase inhibits the body from utilizing vitamin D. while vitamin D3 is needed for brain development and function. This creates a grave problem that these physicians and researchers found, where some of these children experienced slow brain development and/or autism. This is a serious problem and hopefully, the use of nagalase in vaccinations has been stopped. If you have infants who need vaccinating, you might ask the physician or nurse if nagalase is in the vaccination.

Vitamin D3 can also regulate the absorption of calcium and phosphorus. It helps the immune system, growth of the brain, bone, and teeth formation. I suggest if you get little sunshine that you take 125 micro mg (5000 IU), while children under 6 need 50 micro mg. vitamin D3 per day. The recent coronavirus pandemic also brings to light the value of D3 for fighting cancer and virus infections. Cancer dosage: 25,000 IUs for 3-4 months, then 10,000 IUs/day. Coronavirus dosage; 10 to 15,000 IUs./ day, with vitamin C.

The Importance of Iodine

Lack of iodine is considered to be one of the most important causes of health damage in the world. According to the World Health Organization, it affects over two billion people worldwide. Dr. David Brownstein, an authority on iodine, states that over 52 million people in the U.S. have an iodine deficiency. This accounts for one out of every seven people in the U.S. Iodine is needed in over 30 reactions in the body.

Pregnant and breast-feeding mothers have a special need for iodine. It helps in the brain development of the fetus and is vital after the child is born. Most adults do not realize that a lack of iodine is a health hazard for themselves and their families. It can create many health problems.

Researchers are finding that iodine deficiency (hypothyroidism) is the cause of many problems including brain damage and autism. Giving children iodine for brain development is as important as giving them vitamin D3. Other iodine deficiencies are 1. Thyroid enlargement (goiter). 2. Mental retardation in young infants. 3. Depression, weight gain, brittle nails, and hair loss. 4. Anxiety, fatigue, and emotional disturbances. 5. Tiredness and slow brain function.

Between birth and one year, a child should have 110 mcg to 130 mcg of iodine. The adult recommendation is around 500 – 1000 mcg daily. You cannot harm yourself by taking too much iodine, but you should check with your physician about the individual dosage.

Iodine comes from sea kelp. Seaweed, fish, iodine deposits, and bottled iodine. Lately, people have found that Himalayan salt not only provides iodine but is suppose to have over 80 naturally occurring trace minerals. It may be wise to buy Himalayan pink salt, sea salt, or kelp salt. It is rumored that some companies have substituted bromine for iodine in some salts because it is cheaper. For more information, you may look up Dr. David Brownstein, pink salt, or sea salt on your computer.

ELECTROMAGNETIC
GOOD DIET VOLTAGE
(pH) 6.2-6.8

NUTRITIONAL VALUE
[6]

[100]
(100 – 50 Ionic)

Magnesium, Selenium and Chromiuml

The human body uses sixty-seven different minerals to perform its millions of cellular reactions daily. Of these minerals, several are extremely vital to a person's health. Calcium, magnesium, selenium, and chromium are four of these important minerals. Dr. Carolyn Dean says that magnesium is by far the most important mineral in the human body. I disagree!! I think calcium is the most important because you cannot even have a body if you do not have a body without bones, teeth, cartilage, tissue, cells, and very importantly, your steady heart rhythm. However, that discussion is still debatable because you need all of the sixty-seven minerals to complete your daily body cell and organ requirements.

Magnesium is calcium's most important helper and is needed in more than 300 cellular reactions. Some of the most important are: 1. Needed for healthy blood and blood pressure. 2. Helps control blood sugar. 3. It helps maintain and is involved in cellular reactions with calcium. 4. Helps in the cellular reactions in the blood vessels and heart. 5. Helps control fatigue. 6. Helps prevent premature aging, etc.

A magnesium deficiency will help create HBP, Muscle cramps, fatigue, and many other unhealthy body symptoms and reactions. The daily body requirement for magnesium is about 400 mg. Magnesium citrate is a good form of magnesium supplement and is easily absorbable.

Selenium

Why is selenium so important? It is because of the antioxidant properties, plus having a key role in body metabolism. Humans usually get enough selenium in the diet, but people with arthritis and other autoimmune diseases may need to take supplement selenium because it helps in reducing inflammation and radical cell damage. If using supplements, it may be wise not to exceed 100 micro mg

Chromium

Chromium has antioxidant properties plus has a key role in body metabolism. Humans usually get enough chromium in their diet, but if they have diabetes, it is wise to take supplemental chromium, as it helps to control blood sugar. Otherwise, the body needs very little chromium. Suggested dosage: 200 mcmg. a day.

ELECTROMAGNETIC
GOOD DIET VOLTAGE
(pH) 6.2-6.8

NUTRITIONAL VALUE
[6]

[95]

(100 – 50 Ionic)

Xylitol, Honey, Coconut Sweetener, and Dark Chocolate

Xylitol, honey, and coconut sweetener are all good substitutes for sugar, plus are much better for your health. People with cancer are instructed not to eat anything with sugar and carbohydrates in it, as cancer cells love sugar, carbohydrates, and low oxygen. The use of xylitol (from birch trees) and coconut sweetener is much preferred for cancer patients, but even they are cautioned to use it sparingly.

Now for the good part. Dark chocolate is one of the best foods you can eat. It has an incredible amount of health benefits. Some nutritionists and physicians advocate eating dark chocolate three to four times a week. For starters, it has a high concentration of minerals. Especially important are magnesium, phosphate, and iron.

But the next reason makes chocolate a superfood. It is excellent for your heart and blood pressure. It improves blood flow and lowers your risk of strokes, heart attacks, and blood clots. It helps the brain as well as lowers stress. It also encourages the brain to release endorphins, making you and the rest of the players feel happier. It helps control blood sugar, is a mild stimulant, and full of vitamins and minerals.

One caution: I know what you were thinking when you went down the candy counter. Do not let your inner genie sway you from getting the right chocolate that is good for you. Remember, 80 to 95% dark chocolate, not chocolate candy.

ELECTROMAGNETIC GOOD DIET VOLTAGE (pH) 6.2-6.8   **NUTRITIONAL VALUE [6]**   **[95]**

(100 – 50 Ionic)

Farm Raised Poultry and eggs

Economics and convenience have forced the poultry industry to raise many kinds of poultry in cages. Pen raised poultry and eggs are not nearly as good for you as farm-raised poultry and eggs. Pen raising exposes them to GMO corn, hormones, and antibiotics, which create way too much omega 6 fat, toxins, antibiotics, and contaminants in the poultry meat and eggs.

Farm-raised organic poultry is much better than regular poultry but is hard to find in regular grocery stores. Some stores have organic farm-raised eggs in the poultry section. Meat stores usually have farm-raised beef, pork, poultry, and eggs, but farm-raised meat may be hard to find in some areas.

If you have the opportunity to obtain farm-raised poultry and other meat, you will reap the rewards. It is much healthier and contains far less fat, no hormones, no antibiotics, few toxins, and has a much better muscle to fat ratio.

It may be a good idea to take the skins off of any pen-raised chickens before frying or baking. Also, raw eggs or lightly boiled or poached eggs are much better for you than heavy cooking or hard-boiling.

if you live in the city, you might strike a deal with a country's organic farmer. Your smog for their sunshine, farm-raised chickens, and eggs

ELECTROMAGNETIC GOOD DIET VOLTAGE (pH) 6.2-6.4

NUTRITIONAL VALUE

[6]

[100]

(100 – 50 Ionic)

Turmeric (curry), Ginger

Hidden deep in the turmeric plant's roots is an extraordinary compound (spice) called curcumin (curry). It has a unique ability to block an enzyme that causes intestinal and body cell inflammation.

Some people have called turmeric [powder, curry, and capsules} the greatest free radical scavenger of the century. It combats free radical body cell damage. Free radicals (body cell molecules that have lost one or more electrons) are the cause of cellular inflammation. One example is the swelling and enlargement of the joints of arthritic patients, another is the plaque buildup inside of the arteries. Turmeric has been credited with at least twenty five great health benefits.

Besides fighting free radical cell damage, some of the most important benefits are 1. Helps remove plaque from blood vessels, especially in the brain. 2. Promotes brain function. 3. Helps create a better and healthier bacteria environment in the intestines. 4. It helps in the formation of and to strengthen the immune system. 5. Breaks down beta-amyloid plaque in the brain. 6. Helps in the digestion of food. 7. Lowers blood pressure, 8. Helps prevent heart attacks and strokes. 9. Helps prevent intestinal inflammation and leaky gut. etc.

A person can sprinkle turmeric or curry on food, mix it in food and/or drinks, make or buy the capsules. To save the cost of buying turmeric capsules or pills, a person can buy the turmeric powder and make their turmeric capsules at a greatly reduced price. At most drug stores they have number 2 capsules, and capsule maker forms. (or you can get them online) You can make 50 capsules at a time with turmeric powder, which you can get at the health food store. The capsule maker can be obtained from Amazon. The cost is usually around 0.15 cents per capsule, and are not hard to make. My suggestion is to take two to three turmeric and ginger capsules a day

ELECTROMAGNETIC
GOOD DIET VOLTAGE
(pH) 6.6-7.2

NUTRITIONAL VALUE
[6]

[100]

(100 – 50 Ionic)

173

[15]   **Electromagnetic Food**   **Card**
Nutrition   **#28**
Value

Oxygen, Exercise, L-Arginine, and Gingko Biloba

Why is oxygen so important to your health? Because oxygen is one of the most life-giving elements and we cannot live without it. The more oxygen we get, in most cases, the more energy we have and the healthier we stay. The second reason is that our bodies were meant to move. Our early ancestors were on the move all of the time. They had to move (exercise) not only to find food and shelter but also to escape from harm, make shelters, and find firewood.

Most of us do not exercise enough and do not realize how important it is. If a person can exercise about 15 to 30 minutes a day, in most cases it will be very beneficial. Athletic trainers are now saying that hard exercise for ten to fifteen minutes a day will be enough to stimulate your circulatory system and keep you healthy. If you can't use hard exercise, even moderate exercise will help your lungs and body increase the oxygen in your system.

Many older people cannot do strenuous exercises. Walking, sports, swimming, or exercising on machines will still help them a lot. Many supplements will help increase the oxygen in your system. Some of these are L-arginine, resveratrol, turmeric, astaxanthin, and Ginkgo Biloba. Most of them contain nitric oxide, which stimulates and will widen the blood vessels which allows more blood and oxygen to get to the body cells. Nitric oxide stimulates the release of insulin which helps in the digestion of blood sugar. It also helps in lowering high blood pressure, angina, migraine headaches, erectile dysfunction, and much more. Taking a nitric oxide supplement may be very beneficial for your health. Here are some of the great benefits of exercise and nitric oxide supplements: 1. Keeps the blood vessels, muscles and body cells limber plus keeps the heart healthier. 2. Enlarges, Improves, and keeps the lung capacity (oxygen receptors) available to receive more oxygen and transfer it into the blood. Here are some of the great benefits of exercise and nitric oxide supplements:

1. Keeps the blood vessels, muscles and body cells limber plus keeps the heart healthier.

2. Enlarges, Improves, and keeps the lung capacity (oxygen receptors) available to receive more oxygen and transfer it into the blood.

3. Regular exercise helps control weight as a general rule.

4. Stretching enhances flexibility and is important for good posture. It improves balance and helps co-ordination plus reduces the chance of injuries.

5. Improves endurance, strength, and muscle tone.

6. Increases or maintains muscle volume if you use more than simple exercises and spend more than fifteen minutes.

7. Improves self-confidence and quality of life.

8. It increases endorphins and makes you feel better.

ELECTROMAGNETIC GOOD DIET VOLTAGE (pH) 6.8-7.4

NUTRITIONAL VALUE [15]

[100]

(100 – 50 Ionic)

Tomatoes, Salsa and Tomato Sauce

People have been growing and eating tomatoes for a long time. Tomatoes have some good benefits in the ingredients, lycopene, as well as vitamin C, and several other vitamins and minerals. However, in recent research, scientists have found that tomatoes have an ingredient that can cause inflammation of the intestines. Those substances are called "lectins." Lectins are more prevalent in raw tomatoes than other lectin foods. Cooking lectins seems to help greatly in reducing the lectins. Drying tomatoes also seems to reduce the lectins when the tomatoes are then soaked and cooked.

Some other foods that contain lectins are peanuts, grains, beans, potatoes, and cashews. Cooking all of these foods seems to reduce the lectins, and moderate use should give a person little harm. Dr. Steven Gundry has said that lectins can inflame the intestinal wall which will lead to "a leaky gut." Leaky gut from lectins, toxins, candida fungus, and intestinal inflammation will enable protein molecules and small food particles to escape into the blood. Leaky gut is one of the major causes of disease including autoimmune and many other serious illnesses such as ulcers, HBP, diabetes, heart disease, candida infestation, rheumatoid arthritis, asthma, leukocytosis, brain disorders, cancer plus others.

However, the author does not think that you should lay off of lectins. Recent literature states that lectins are not as serious as Dr. Gundry thinks.

Tomatoes, tomato sauce, salsa, and other cooked tomato products, mixed with other foods have a smaller amount of lectins. They also have some good health benefits, so I feel that if eaten in moderate or small amounts, they will cause little harm. Since tomatoes and these tomato products mixed with other foods have been eaten for hundreds of years, the consumption should not be a concern unless a person eats a large number of raw tomatoes or excess cooked varieties of tomatoes and other lectins.

ELECTROMAGNETIC GOOD DIET VOLTAGE (pH) 5.8-6.6	NUTRITIONAL VALUE [5]	[65] (100 – 50 Ionic) (50-0 Cationic)

177

Milk, Milk Products, and Cheeses

Everyone likes milk. It is essential for babies (especially important in mother's milk). Milk contains a lot of protein and calcium, plus other vitamins and minerals.

FDA, milk producers, and retailers have not been honest about advertising milk. When it comes to nutrition, pasteurizing may keep children and adults from getting certain diseases such as brucellosis, but heating milk destroys more than 40 different antibodies, milk fats, and other nutrients.

Raw human milk is recommended by all pediatricians and physicians and is a great starter for all children. Most pediatricians say the recommended time that a baby should be on mother's milk for one and years or more. The antibodies, milk fats, protein, calcium, and other nutrients provide protection and nutrition the baby cannot get from cow's milk.

Feeding a young baby pasteurized cow's milk is not helping the baby and is hard for the baby to digest. Pasteurized milk is not very healthy for adults either. Lately, some pediatricians are recommending almond milk over pasteurized cow's milk. The only drawback is concerning calcium, but if babies and people eat a lot of vegetables, fruit, and canned fish and supplements, they should get plenty of calcium.

Most powdered milk is pasteurized, so the antibodies and many nutrients are gone. Also, other forms of pasteurized milk maintain the same properties as regular milk.

Cheeses

Most cheeses are made from non pasteurized milk and are good for you. White cheeses are more nutritious than colored cheeses. Since most cheeses are not pasteurized it is a big plus in the digestion department, plus they contain calcium, protein, milk fats, and other vitamins and nutrients. However, if the cheese is pasteurized, the nutritious value of all pasteurized cheese products will bring the nutrition value way down.

ELECTROMAGNETIC GOOD DIET VOLTAGE (pH) 6.0-6.8

NUTRITIONAL VALUE [5]

[60]

(100 – 50 Ionic)

Butter

A good piece of rye toast with genuine butter tastes mighty good. Butter is a dairy product containing up to 80 percent saturated butterfat. It is solid when chilled but softens at room temperature. It consists of butterfat, milk proteins, and some other nutrients.

Some butter has salt added and will state so on the container. Other butter may not have salt. Garlic is sometimes added for flavor. Butter consists of triglycerides, glycol, and fatty acids. It can become rancid when left in hot areas for a length of time.

Even though it is mostly saturated fat, it is a good cooking fat, second only to coconut and hemp oils. Many cooks in famous restaurants use it for their cooking. Butter contains a substance called butyric acid. It breaks down into butyrate. Butyrate inhibits colon tumors and helps prevent colon cancer, and also helps in the reduction of type 2 diabetes. A small amount is also needed in the transfer of nutrients from the blood into the body cells.

Butter's advantage puts it far ahead of margarine on the captain's table. Margarine is an imitation butter that was invented when requested by Emperor Napoleon. It is water in a fat emulsion containing tiny drops of water. Its main ingredient is an omega-6 (dead) fat from vegetable oil and has no food value. I feel that butter is a far healthier fat than margarine.

If you are using margarine you might look upon your computer the beneficial contents of butter and the disadvantages of margarine. I think you would choose butter.

ELECTROMAGNETIC
GOOD DIET VOLTAGE
(pH) 6.2-6.4

NUTRITIONAL VALUE
[5]

[95]

(100 – 50 Ionic)

(50 – 0 Ionic)

Canned Fruits and Vegetable

Canned vegetables and fruit have been around since the 1600s. Before people had refrigerators, canning was a very good way to save food for a later day, plus canning saved a lot of the vitamins, minerals, and enzymes. Even today, most of us depend on canned vegetables, berries, and fruit but unfortunately, the glass jar has for the most part been replaced by the can.

How do canned foods compare with fresh natural, or frozen vegetables and fruit? Canned foods still have much nutrition, but lose about 40 percent to 50 percent of the vital vitamins, enzymes, and minerals that are in the raw fresh varieties. This is still much better than eating food that has no electromagnetic food value at all, such as oils on the grocery shelf, sugar products, red meat, and deep=fried French fries, chips, and other carbohydrates. Some of the advantages of canned foods are

1. They are completely natural and most still have a lot of fiber.

2. If you can put them in jars or cans and cook them yourself you can put in the desired spices, salt, and sugar with no preservatives.

3. Commercially canned foods, especially fruits, have sometimes too much sugar, sometimes preservatives, and maybe too much salt for a conservative health convert.

4. Most canned fruits and vegetables are good and healthy products. They keep a long time if kept cool or cold.

5. They are very stable and keep the electromagnetic value, although it may be much less than fresh vegetables and fruit.

6. They are very good when a person is in a desolate location and they cannot get to a grocery store or place where they can get fresh vegetables and fruit.

7. Some vegetables and fruit, when bought in commercial cans, may have preservatives, be overcooked, have too much sugar, and are found to have the cans lined with plastic to preserve the taste. It is hard to know unless you read the labels, and inspect the cans after you have poured out the contents. Glass is the best for canning. Watch out for too much sugar and sweeteners in fruits.

ELECTROMAGNETIC
GOOD DIET VOLTAGE
(pH) 5.8-6.6

NUTRITIONAL VALUE
[5]

[65]

(100 – 50 Ionic)

Bananas, Mangos, and Kiwis

There has been a lot of negative publicity about bananas. The talk is that bananas, especially when ripe, have a lot of sugar. Sugar is one of nutrition's "bad monsters." However, bananas, mangos, and kiwi when not overripe are very affordable, and nutritious fruits. My suggestion about bananas and mangos is to not buy a large amount all at one time when extra days will ripen them fast.

1. High in fiber; bananas, kiwi, and mangos help to regulate your digestive system and improve regularity

2. These fruits boost energy. They are much better than regular breakfast cereals, cinnamon rolls, and other carbohydrates, eaten for breakfast.

3. They all have a substance, tryptophan, which produces serotonin, amino acids, and great neurotransmitter.

4. They all boost energy, have many nutrients, and are much better than energy bars

5. They have high potassium and phosphate, needed to control blood pressure and heart disease

6. Bananas have magnesium, which works with calcium to strengthen bones

7. Mangos, kiwis, and bananas help maintain kidney function with their phenolic compounds

I feel that the overall advantages of these fruits outweigh the disadvantages. I suggest that you refrain from eating these fruits if very ripe

ELECTROMAGNETIC GOOD DIET VOLTAGE (pH) 5.8-6.6	NUTRITIONAL VALUE [4]	[65] (100 – 50 Ionic) (50 – 0 Cationic)

185

Vegetables, Cooked the Optimum Time

Nutritionists tell us that steamed, boiled, or broiled vegetables need to be done but not too well done or overcooked. When they are overcooked they lose a lot of their vitamins, enzymes, minerals, and amino acids. In a report by the "Journal of Food Science," vegetables are very heat sensitive and easy to overcook. When they are, the nutrients that are heat sensitive are quickly destroyed.

But wait! Boiling or steaming some vegetables for more than four to six minutes increases the nutrients and antioxidants. Carrots (containing beta carotene), maybe be cooked for twelve to fourteen minutes, and tomatoes (containing lycopene) may be cooked eight to ten minutes while still retaining their antioxidants. Cooking also reduces the number of lectins. Prolonged heating of most vegetables decreases the nutrients and antioxidants as the heating continues.

Some important cooking facts:

1. Most vegetables still have a lot of nutrients when cooked in under six minutes

2. Stir-frying maintains nutrients much like steaming and/or boiling

3. When cooking carrots, beets, and potatoes with other vegetables, cook them for about six to eight minutes before adding the other, softer vegetables

4. Cooking and eating too many potatoes will increase your carbohydrate intake. Carbohydrates turn to sugar in your digestive system.

5. Cooking, steaming, and boiling vegetables will lose much of the vitamin C and anthocyanins, while they enhance vitamins A, D, K, and E

Boil wisely, my friend, but not too much. Lightly boiled vegetables are a great way to keep your electromagnetic ionic body cells happy, much better than any refined or other processed foods, but not a good as fresh vegetables.

ELECTROMAGNETIC GOOD DIET VOLTAGE (pH) 6.2-6.8

NUTRITIONAL VALUE [4]

[75]
(100 – 50 Ionic)
(100 – 50 Cationic)

Foods from Flour, Bread, Breakfast Cereal and Pizza

Since the discovery that seeds of grain could be ground into flour to make bread, it has been one of the oldest foods used on earth. It is consumed in just about every country in the world. Many cultures of people have relied on different forms of bread for many centuries. Most cultures do not just eat bread alone, for many other nutrients are needed to maintain their health.

Most grains and flour products contain carbohydrates, minerals, some protein, B vitamins, iron, selenium, and fiber. It is a very good food source but has drawbacks when people overeat bread and flour products or add substances like sugar, preservatives, and coloring which is not good for your health.

Bread has many uses, and millions of people break and eat bread in churches all over the world. Other cultures use it for religious rituals and secular events. The English word "lord," is derived from an Anglo Saxon word, "bread keepers." Bread, breakfast food, and pizzas are three of the most popular foods purchased and eaten in the United States. Forty to fifty percent of households all over the country have breakfast cereal, mush, and or toast every morning. The reason is that these foods are easy and fast to prepare. Bread with butter, and cereals with milk, sugar, honey, sweets, berries, or other fruit, make a fast and supposedly healthy meal. However, there are drawbacks.

Recent research has shown that bread, breakfast cereal, pasta, pizza, and other flour products may not be as healthful as previously thought. All nutrition of grains is in the husk. The inside of the grain has no food value. Most people do not realize that certain other grains have a lot more nutrients than wheat. Rye has 12 times more nutrients than wheat and six times more nutrients than oats. Rye is a much better choice than oats and wheat in bread and mush. Rolled rye can be bought at the health food store and maybe a better choice than oats in heated breakfast cerea

Wheat flour also contains an unusual substance called amylopectin-A, which in tests has been shown to "spike' your blood sugar. Besides glycolysis, there are hundreds of studies about the amount of gluten in wheat flour. Many studies

Excess gluten will cause toxins, inflammation of the intestines, and contribute to candida infestation in your gut. Excess wheat and oat flour in your gut also alter the body collagen, which produces wrinkles and sagging skin. Over time, excess consumption can also increase a person's weight.

I hope that this information is not ruining your day. Some grain products in moderation or better yet used sparingly should not be harmful to your health. However, these products in excess, or combined with other added sugar (glucose), preservatives, flavorings, etc., have many health drawbacks. They can cause weight gain, gut inflammation, leaky gut, and radical body cell damage. My suggestion: Eat carbohydrates sparingly. The sugar (glucose) factor is a big problem. A raw, fruit berry, nut, and melon, cottage cheese with flaxseed oil, and electromagnetic breakfast without cereal or toast are great. A diet with low sugar and carbohydrates is a great step toward more energy, better electromagnetic ionic metabolism, better health, and maybe a longer life. You might also consider Rye bread.

ELECTROMAGNETIC GOOD DIET VOLTAGE (pH) 5.8-6.6	NUTRITIONAL VALUE [4]	[40] (100 – 50 Ionic) (50 – 0 Ionic)

[4]   **Non-Electromagnetic**   **Card**
Nutrition   **Food**   **#36**
Value

Coffee Additives, Non-Dairy Creamer, Cream, Almond and Soy Milk

What's in your coffee? We probably would be better off if we drank coffee without anything. Yet millions of people like to put some "goodie' in their coffee. Non-dairy creamer was introduced to coffee drinkers in 1989. Since then it has become a household name and comes in several varieties, plus a dry, sugar variation. In the U.S., many creamers are made with hydrogenated fat, water, sugar carrageenan, vegetable oil, mono and diglycerides, dipotassium sulfate, and preservatives. The European variety is made without hydrogenated fat. Hydrogenated fat is linked to HBP and heart disease. Most creamers contain glucose, partially hydrogenated soybean oil, milk protein, stabilizer, sodium citrate, and other ingredients. Some articles say that the other ingredients are partially hydrogenated vegetable oil (trans fat).

Cream has always been a staple additive for coffee. Cream, is a much better choice than glucose added coffee additives, although it contains milk fats. I suggest refraining from using large amounts of cream. Almond milk also has some drawbacks but is better than creamer or coffee mate for a coffee additive. Almond milk contains a small amount of glucose, but most of the other ingredients seem to contain healthier nutrients, including calcium, magnesium, and other vitamins. Although almond milk has some setbacks, it is kidney-friendly, as it does not have milk protein and is low in potassium and phosphate. People with kidney disease need to restrict potassium and phosphate. Almond milk is also high in calcium, which helps in raising bone density levels. It also is a good substitute for pasteurized milk and is lactose-free, which helps people with high cholesterol and/or heart disease.

Nine things that are added to your coffee may be very concerning.

1. Sugar (glucose)

2. Stevia

3. Aspertame

4. Sucralose

5. Powdered Cream

6. Corn Syrup

7. Saccharin

8. Hydrogenated Oils

9. Coffee-mate

If you want an additive, a small amount of honey, cream or almond milk may be your best bet.

ELECTROMAGNETIC GOOD DIET VOLTAGE (pH) 6.2-6.8

NUTRITIONAL VALUE [4]

[45]

(50 – 0 Cationic)

Ice Cream, Shakes, Sodas, Whipped Cream

Ice cream is something that it is hard to say no to. It is a frozen, sweetened food served as a snack, cone, dish, frozen dairy, sherbet, or ice cream bar. It contains 17 – 22 percent sugar in most forms. To preserve a person's health, people shouldn't make a daily habit of eating ice cream or ice cream products.

Ice cream has been around for many years. It was found in China about 200 B. C. The many forms make it one of the most popular desserts, with syrups, fruits, berries, cakes, pies, shakes, cones, and just plain ice cream. I suggest you do not regularly eat ice cream, because of the sugar and cream content. People with heart disease, diabetes, high blood pressure, and cancer should eat it very sparingly, or not at all.

Ice Cream Sodas and Shakes

Ice cream sodas and shakes have been around since the 1800s. Since first introduced they have made it all around the world. In Canada, ice cream sodas are called "cream sodas," while in Latin America sodas are called, "red pop." In South Africa and Zimbabwe, ice cream soda is called "sparlette" or a "green ambulance." However, with any name, Ice cream sodas and shakes are still high sugar food and should be treated the same as ice cream.

Whipped Cream

Whipped cream becomes a colloid when whipped. Air bubbles are trapped in it, producing a fluffy mixture. If the mixing is continued, the cream will turn to butter. Lower fat cream (less than 35 percent butter-fat, does not mix well and produces a mixture with less foam. Whipped cream is often flavored with sugar, vanilla, flavoring, or even honey. Outside of the fat content, most whipped cream may be worth satisfying the palate once in a while. Surprisingly, some varieties of whipped cream are mixed with nitrous oxide, which is good for you.

ELECTROMAGNETIC GOOD DIET VOLTAGE (pH) 5.8-6.6

NUTRITIONAL VALUE [4]

[20]

(50 - 0 Cationic)

Potatoes, Sweet Potatoes, and Yams

The very first potatoes were found in southern Peru and northwest Bolivia, around 7,000 – 10,000 years ago. There are about 1,000 different varieties of potatoes. They are grown all over the world. China and India lead the world in potato output with more than 37 percent of the total production.

Raw potatoes contain many vitamins and minerals in small amounts. They are two percent protein and a rich source of vitamins, B6 and C. Potatoes have a high glycemic index because of the starch. The raw, young sprouts of potatoes are very nutritious. Many people who are on a diet should eat skimpy portions, as the high glycemic index changes the starch to glucose in a person's digestive tract. Boiling or frying reduces vitamins and enzymes. It also reduces the lectins, which in large amounts are known to harm the intestinal lining of the gut.

As potatoes mature, several changes occur. They develop a mildly toxic compound known as glycol-alkaloids. This can be observed when exposure to light increases glycol-alkaloids and the tops of the potatoes turn green before digging. Cooking decreases glycol-alkaloids. Cooked potatoes are much more nutritious than eating raw.

Most red and colored potatoes have more carotenoids and polyphenols, which makes them more nutritious than white potatoes. Potatoes have lectins, glycol-alkaloids, and starch. They also turn to glucose in your intestines. As good as they taste, you shouldn't put them on your no-fly list. Enjoy potatoes, but I suggest you do not use them in excess, deep-fried, or as a steady diet. Holidays should not be passed without them.

Sweet potatoes and yams (very nutritious) belong to the bindweed and/or morning glory family. They are only a distant relative of regular potatoes. The young leaves are also eaten as greens. Sweet potatoes with white or yellow flesh are less sweet than potatoes, have red or pink skins, plus more nutrients.

Sweet potatoes are rich in starch, complex carbohydrates, dietary fiber, beta carotene, carotenoids, micronutrients including vitamins B2, B6, A, and manganese.

Yams are equivalent to sweet potatoes in nutrients plus are very high in potassium. The nutritional value is higher than many other species of potatoes and grains. Although potatoes, sweet potatoes, and yams have lectins, they are good food if not eaten too often or deep-fried. They are very good for the holidays.

ELECTROMAGNETIC
GOOD DIET VOLTAGE
(pH) 6.2-6.8

NUTRITIONAL VALUE
[3]

[25]

(50 – 0 Cationic)

Beer, Wine, Champagne, and Hard Alcohol Drinks

Alcoholic drinks are a very common thing in the U.S. and the U.K. They are consumed all over the world. Beer, wine, and champagne are fermented drinks. Champagne is a double fermented drink and many alternative cancer physicians in Europe serve and claim a little champagne is good for cancer patients. I have mentioned before about fermented foods, and feel that they are a benefit for a person's health. Most red wines, some white wines, and most champagnes have polyphenols and catechins. Moderate use is supposed to be a help in the prevention of HBP, heart disease, and supposedly slender waistlines. That is if social drinking does not become a habitual entity.

Beer has been made and consumed all over the world since the 1400s. In the early ages, it was the most bacteria free drink in most countries. It took the place of water in many places, since most waters were not pure, while beer was without dangerous bacteria. Beer in moderate usage does little harm to a person's health. However, excess consumption may cause obesity. Overzealous drinking of beer may have some effect in providing many excess calories.

Hard liquor is a term used in North America which is different from fermented alcohol. It is distilled from many ingredients into different forms of alcoholic drinks. Distilled drinks are made from raw materials which include grain, potatoes, hops, rice, cactus, vegetables, berries, or fruit that can be fermented and distilled. Hard drinks in small amounts may produce some cardiovascular benefits. However, short term effects of heavy consumption can lead to intoxication, dehydration, impaired vision, neural confusion, and underlined uncontrolled movements. Long term effects are not very healthful and can lead to many severe problems. The problems depend on the amount and frequency of alcoholic consumption. Long term, chronic use can lead to cirrhosis of the liver, pancreatic, and kidney problems. In the U.S., overconsumption of alcohol, mostly hard liquor, contributes to about 90,000 deaths each year. Worldwide, deaths from alcohol in 2019 stacked up to 3.3 million people.

ELECTROMAGNETIC
GOOD DIET VOLTAGE
(pH) 5.5-6.2

NUTRITIONAL VALUE
[3]

[25]

(50 – 0 Cationic)

Energy Drinks, Energy Bars

Energy drinks are the fastest-growing category in the soft drink market. Some of the most popular are: Red Bull, V Energy, Powerade, Energy Edge, Five Hour Energy and Enviga. Most of the hype and use is because of hectic lifestyles, long working hours, and high temperatures.

Drinking more than one energy drink a day may put a strain on the liver, because of the high dose of niacin and caffeine. While most energy drinks do not have as much caffeine as in many coffee shops, they are still heavily sweetened with sucrose and/or glucose. These substances, in excess, can affect your adrenal glands which in turn affect your thyroid hormones. Many people drink four to seven energy drinks a day. Any excess amount may cause the following problems: Addiction to sugar and caffeine, gall bladder overload, niacin overdose, insomnia, and headaches. Some people with excess use of energy drinks have developed hepatitis, caused by toxic liver overload.

What else is inside energy drinks? Some have B vitamins, taurine, an amino acid, goji extract, and beet juice. They may boost your energy but It may be wise to limit your intake.

Energy Bars

Energy bars have become the "must-have energy" solution to people in every workplace and outdoor recreation category. It is a $1.3 billion market in the U.S. There is a sharp difference between energy bars and protein bars. There are good and bad ingredients in both. Protein bars are an entirely different category, but many protein bars have some "cationic foods" inside the wrapper. Some of the best protein bars are Great

Nutrition, Optimum Nutrition, Kind Bars, Zing Nutrition, and Three in One Nutrition.

Some energy and protein bars are healthful, but many have a lot of ingredients that are not. Most bars contain: Corn syrup, palm kernel oil, sucralose, natural flavors, skim milk, peanuts, Splenda, aspartame, caffeine, soy protein, isolate, glycerin, soy, lecithin, excess salt, sucrose, corn syrup, etc

Most of these ingredients are "dead," non-electromagnetic acetic substances. Some of the better-rated bars are Raw Crunch, Yaws, and Raw Revolution. There are more than 50 varieties of all nutrition grades, so please select wisely. You may also be very wise to read the labels.

ELECTROMAGNETIC GOOD DIET VOLTAGE (pH) 5.6-6.2

NUTRITIONAL VALUE [3]

[25]

(50 – 0 Cationic)

Hamburgers, Fish Burgers

Hamburgers are probably the most often eaten meal outside of the home kitchen. They are a delicious meal and taste great. However, they have many drawbacks for the conscientious nutrition advocate.

Hamburgers come in many different variations, most of which are high calories and without a lot of nutrition. Usually, the more that is added, the less nutrition there is in the package. Hamburgers are usually fried in saturated oil, and that is the start of a non-electromagnetic acetic sandwich. They usually have way too much salt which averages 380 mg. The hamburger's total fat is around 18 grams, which is all saturated fat. Sugars and carbohydrates, 15 grams. The cholesterol is about 30 mg, and if you add cheese, you may be able to double that. Unfortunately, hamburgers have very few vitamins, minerals, and good nutrients. It is a shame that more people do not go for good, nutritious, electromagnetic food instead of fast, non-electromagnetic, acetic food.

Fish burgers, if not deep-fried, are comparable to fried hamburgers except with fish there are some good omega 3 fats unless the fish has been in the deep-fried saturated fat for cooking. There is very little difference in the total overall fat content, cholesterol, and salt. As a health food, most fish burgers are way down on the fish-eating scale.

Many people love the idea of a fast, cheap meal and something that fills their stomach and appetite. Most of these people also add a sugared or diet fast drink, and French fries to satisfy their intestinal bacterial cravings for fries and sugar. These foods have very few nutrients and are not good for your health.

Recently, McDonald's, Burger King, Arby's, and Jack in the Box added a salad to their menu. It is a much better nutritious choice for lunch, even if you are in a hurry

ELECTROMAGNETIC
GOOD DIET VOLTAGE
(pH) 5.8-6.2

NUTRITIONAL VALUE
[3]

[15]
(100 – 50 Ionic)
(50-0 Cationic)

Red Meat and Pork

Most everyone loves a great grilled steak or roast. Bacon, ham and eggs, a rack of lamb, baby back ribs, or maybe hamburgers are always popular items for breakfast, lunch and dinner. Even talking about these foods makes a person's mouth water.

Please do not be unhappy with me if I give you some unhappy nutrition advice. For cancer prevention, red meat and pork should be eaten sparingly. Pen-raised beef has about 30 percent interstitial fat, and it is mostly omega 6. Also, if pen-raised and from the grocery store, it probably is intermixed with hormones and antibiotics. The animal may also have been fed with GMO corn and alfalfa, and vaccination toxins. Many of the animals bought from the grocery store are raised in pens with GMO corn, hormones, antibiotics, and other toxins.

Farm-raised beef and pork usually have a better monosaturated fat content without as many omega-six fatty acids, but still enough that the fats plus the acetic cationic contents place the red meat into a low nutrition (acid) category. It is hard to dismiss the fats, but there is also another problem. Your pancreas produces only enough protease enzymes to digest about four ounces of red meat protein Any surplus puts a burden on the liver and gall bladder. The gall bladder is overlooked because it cannot metabolize very much omega-six fat at any one time. It is hard to hear bad news about such good food. However, making a routine habit of red meat may lower your normal pH range and bring it into an acetic, cationic, inflammatory, and radical oxidative cell range. Cancer loves red meat and sugar, all because it loves an acetic body and low oxygen. Wild meat, although acetic, is much better, because it contains much less fat.

I suggest, if you want a healthy preventive cancer diet, that you eat red meat only on special occasions or sparingly. Otherwise, when you do, there is a pancreatic enzyme, wobenzym-N that contains pancreatic enzymes and may help digest the amounts over four ounces or more.

ELECTROMAGNETIC GOOD DIET VOLTAGE (pH) 5.6-6.2

NUTRITIONAL VALUE [3]

[15]

(50-0 Cationic)

Peanuts and Cashews

Peanuts and cashews are legumes that have been grown by man for centuries. They are high in calories. A one-quarter cup having around 600 calories per three ounces. When raw (but not heated) they have monounsaturated fatty acids, especially oleic acid. The nuts increase a person's HDL (good cholesterol) and are a good source of protein. Peanuts also contain resveratrol, a polyphenol antioxidant that has a protective function against cancer, heart, and Alzheimer's disease. Also, they have vitamin E, B vitamins, folate, and many minerals.

With a batting average like that, you would think that peanuts and cashews would be superfoods. I hate to say, but there are some drawbacks. There are two problems with peanuts and cashews and some doctors have said they should be eaten sparingly. They contain high amounts of lectins. Publications have stated that lectins protect these nuts from being attacked by insects and other intruders. Dr. Gundry has also shown, lectins are the cause of intestinal inflammation and leaky gut in the small intestine, However, recent research has shown that lectins are not as damaging as Dr. Gundry has said they are.

Excess lectins have a toxic coating that attacks the intestinal cell wall and causes gut perforations. These gut wall perforations (holes) make a pathway for protein molecules, minute food particles, bad bacteria, and viruses to go directly into your blood. This will result in several diseases including autoimmune disease, Crone's disease, leucocytosis, allergies, and other inflammatory and radical cell damage diseases.

Heating or roasting these nuts reduces the toxins in the lectins, but there are still enough lectins to be aware of. Logic says that you be aware of peanut and cashew lectins, but that millions of Americans eat them every day without severe harm. I suggest that you eat them sparingly, or can substitute them with raw almonds, pecans, walnuts, or Brazil nuts.

ELECTROMAGNETIC
GOOD DIET VOLTAGE
(pH) 6.2-6.4

NUTRITIONAL VALUE
[2]

[10]
(100 – 50 Ionic)
(50-0 Cationic)

All Oils on the Grocery Shelf, except Extra Virgin Olive Oil

All oils on the grocery shelf except extra virgin olive oil, are cooked (boiled) to over 300+ degrees. This enables them to stay on the grocery shelf forever without getting rancid. This process changes the oils dramatically. It changes the oils from a monounsaturated and/or polyunsaturated oil into saturated omega 6 oil. When used for cooking these oils turn into "trans fats" and "mega trans," oils that lose their electromagnetic charge and present a problem that is not good for your health. When they are consumed and digested, they are transferred into the bloodstream. With chronic use of these excess trans fats and mega trans (in salads, frying, or deep frying), the blood can form a substance called homocysteine. Homo cysteine is a blood-clotting agent found in many cancers and is responsible for a person getting sticky blood (rouleaux) or blood that clumps and reduces the flow of oxygen. When these excesses (dead electromagnetic) cooked oils transfer to the body cells they also help restrict oxygen in them. Many cancer doctors believe that "low oxygen" in the body cells makes them more susceptible to heart disease, strokes, heart attacks, and sometimes a mitochondrial cancer hit, or a cell that changes into a cancer cell.

Catherine Shanahan, M. D., a Canadian physician, states that restaurants when using these saturated fry oils (trans fats and mega trans) for deep frying and cooking, "are guilty of causing disease states." These mega trans and trans fats cause a massive imbalance with a person's omega 6 to omega 3 ratio which should be a 2 to 1 or 3 to 1 ratio in a person. But the ratio rapidly changes to a 30 to 1 ratio or even a 50 to 1 ratio in a person's body. This means that when you eat French fries or deep-fried foods, your omega 6 to omega 3 ratio changes rapidly. Dr. Shanahan surveyed 215 patients who had just been admitted to her hospital with a heart attack or stroke. She discovered that 90 percent of these patients had consumed foods with these saturated (dead) vegetable oils in their last 24 hours. This is quite a revelation. These oils are very low (dead oils) on the nutrition scale. They are non-electromagnetic, acetic, extra-low pH oils. I suggest coconut oil, palm oil, or butter for cooking or deep frying.

ELECTROMAGNETIC
GOOD DIET VOLTAGE
(pH) 5.6-6.0

NUTRITIONAL VALUE
[2]

[0]

(50-0 Cationic)

[2]   **Non-Electromagnetic**   **Card**
Nutrition   **Food**   **#45**
Value

Refined Foods

Welcome to the artificial world of refined foods. Many kinds of cereals, roll, and cake companies are probably giving their CEO a raise for great sales these days. Unfortunately, your health is paying for their salaries. These refined foods counteract and neutralize the electromagnetic ionic foods that you eat.

There is a long list of these refined culprits, starting with white flour, soy, sugar, artificial ingredients, preservatives, corn syrup, synthetic dyes, artificial sweeteners, such as aspartame, Splenda, sucralose, plus many other "dead" nutrient refined foods.

The FDA has created another problem. Untruth labels and print. Please don't believe everything you read on the labels. Most of these products are not healthful and they are not as nutritious as they state on the labels.

One sneaky trick these companies play is that they use GMO products in their food. There are now over 30,000 GMO corn and soy products on the market. In most foreign countries they make laws that do not allow GMO products to be sold. Here we not only allow them, but the FDA and the government have prohibited GMO literature on the labels. This is a travesty, as research shows that GMO products have been known to cause cancer and other diseases in rats. Many people even think that some companies have quietly made monetary contributions to the lax GMO and label controls.

I believe that live ionic foods are a great thing for breakfast and much better than cinnamon rolls, breakfast cereal, maple bars, and coffee. Mush made from crushed oats or rye, boiled or raw eggs, cottage cheese,

Flax oil and kefir, avocado, melons, berries, raw fresh almonds, walnuts, pecans, fresh fruit, and rye toast are a much better choice for breakfast than a quick, nonnutritious, and cationic refined food diet. Even milk is not as nutritious as the companies say. By the way, all nutrients in grains are in the husk. Rye flour and rye bread have six times more nutrition than oats and 12 times more nutrition than wheat.

ELECTROMAGNETIC GOOD DIET VOLTAGE (pH) 5.8-6.4

NUTRITIONAL VALUE [2]

[10]

(50 – 0 Cationic)

Pies, Cakes, Cookies, Gelatins, Cinnamon Rolls and Puddings

Everyone loves pies, cookies, cakes, gelatins, cinnamon rolls, puddings, and other sugared desserts. Sadly, candida fungus, parasites, bad bacteria, and cancer viruses love sugar too. The average person in the U.S. eats about 22 teaspoons of sugar each day. This totals up to be about an average of 100 to 120 pounds of sugar per person per year. This is unbelievable, but those are the figures from the National Health Association. That amount of sugar feeds a lot of bad hombres in your digestive tract (biome) and immune system. To make things worse, many refined and processed foods now have so much sugar and/or sugar products that it even confuses the smart grocery shopper.

You may not realize it but even flour, potatoes, and other carbohydrates change to glucose in your digestive tract and body. This adds to the average 22 teaspoons of daily sugar, and that isn't even counted with the daily sugar measurements.

A daily double occurs when your daily diet includes sugars with red meat, high carbohydrates, and saturated (dead, non-electromagnetic) vegetable oils. This combination, if consumed often, is a probable cesspool where your small intestines may invite excess candida fungus, bad bacteria, possible parasites, and other nasty guests that ruin your energy, health, girth, and longevity. It is very hard to say, "no, thank you," when offered a tasty prepared dessert. However, most hosts will not be offended if you say you have been laying off of the sugar lately because of your stomach, or ask for a very small portion.

Other tips are

1. Pass up all sugared foods on the grocery shelf when you go shopping.

2. If eating out, try to have mostly lunches that contain limited or no sugar.

3. Try to keep no foods containing sugar in your house.

4. Stay away from diet and sugared soda pop.

5. Substitute dressings and other toppings with cottage cheese, yogurt, coconut sugar, xylitol sugar, or honey.

ELECTROMAGNETIC GOOD DIET VOLTAGE (pH) 5.8-6.2

NUTRITIONAL VALUE [2]

[10]

(50-0 Cationic)

GMO (Genetically Modified) Soy and Corn Products

One of the biggest farm and food rip-offs in history is happening right here in the United States. That is the rumored unethical acts of the FDA, some pesticide companies, and the U.S. government. The rumor is that compensation is passed back and forth between these pesticide companies, the lobbyists, and the FDA. This is a travesty, and the American citizens are the losers. There are more than 30,000 GMO corn and soy and maybe more food products on our grocery shelves, that we do not know about or are on the way.

Research has proven that GMO products have caused cancer in rats, and it is suspected that they also can cause cancer in humans. Most foreign governments (more than 30) have banned the use of GMO products for human consumption. Yet in the U.S. some pesticide and food companies keep cranking out GMO modified food products. Our government keeps saying that GMO labels are not needed. I suggest that since most of the GMO products are hard to distinguish or are not labeled, that a person raises a garden or buy organic products as much as they can, or eat corn and soy products very sparingly.

Genetically modifying plants is a process where herbicides are genetically engineered into the genes of the plants to make them insect and pesticide- resistant. Also, many crops are sprayed with GMO herbicides, not only to kill noxious weeds but later, to also dry the grain and corn. We have been told that roundup is one of those herbicides. Roundup is not good for anyone's health and many people are saying that it should be banned altogether.

Two things you can do: 1. Write or call your congressmen or senators, to let them know you are against genetically modified plants and food. 2. Buy organic whenever you can, especially corn and soy products. All of these organic products will thank your tummy, liver, intestines, body cells, and brain.

ELECTROMAGNETIC
GOOD DIET VOLTAGE
(pH) 6.2-6.4

NUTRITIONAL VALUE
[2]

[0]
(100 – 50 Ionic)
(50 - 0 Cationic)

Cooking Oils, Margarine, Lard, Shortening and Oil Sprays

These saturated oils (all on the grocery shelf except extra virgin olive oil), have been heated to 300 degrees at the processing facility before they are put on the grocery shelf. Processors did not heat oils when oils were first made for cooking, but they would turn rancid when left on the grocery shelf at room temperatures. Because of loss of revenue, grocery store and oil processors started heating these oils to keep them on the shelves until sold. Heating these oils destroys the electromagnetic ionic charge, making them a cationic (dead) oil. They not only have no energy but create an "acid body state" causing many adverse abnormalities. toxins and diseases in your body. The problem arises because many people and most restaurants use these cheap oils for deep frying and frying their foods. They many times also use these oils over and over, creating "transfats" and "mega trans," a serious form of harmful oil. Continued chronic use of these oils can create several forms of disease states. Coupled with red meat and sugar, they can become even greater disease makers and can be attributed to serious diseases including heart disease, and cancer mentioned previously.

When people have Inflammatory toxins, leaky gut, arthritis, high blood pressure, heart disease, poor immune system, candida, parasites, allergies, leucocytosis, and many other ailments, most can be traced back to one or all of these three mean culprits. Excess sugar, red meat, and dead oils may also be triggers in diabetes, strokes, heart attacks, restricted insulin, and many think, the cause of cancer. Recent research has shown that eating deep-fried foods, including French fries, spikes your omega six to omega 3 ratio from normal 2 : 1 or 3 : 1, to 40 : 1 or even 50 : 1. This is enough of a short rise (spike) in ratios to trigger a heart attack or stroke if a person has heart disease, high blood pressure, and "sticky " homocysteine blood or artery plaque.

If cooking, I suggest coconut oil, palm oil, or butter. They are saturated oils that do not have a large molecular change. I also suggest you go extremely light on all oil fried foods, including donuts, bacon, French fries, and deep-fried foods.

ELECTROMAGNETIC
GOOD DIET VOLTAGE
(pH) 5.6-6.2

NUTRITIONAL VALUE
[1]

[-5]

(50 – -5 Cationic)

Sugar, Candy, Glucose, Corn Syrup, and Fructose

Are 22 teaspoons of sugar a day is a little bit much? This is the average amount of sugar and sugar product consumption, per day for every man, woman, and child, in America. The average person consumes up to 100 to 120 pounds of these goodies per year in the U.S.A. One of the problems is the brain addiction cravings for candy and hidden sugars in most of the refined and processed foods.

Believe it or not, your intestinal bacteria communicate with your brain and say, "feed me, feed me." Refined sugars, candy, corn syrup, and glucose products are some of the worst for sugar addiction. They are the most nutritional (dead) foods a person can consume. They not only provide many unwanted calories but are very acetic and change your blood and body cells to a very cationic non-electromagnetic state. That is just the start of the disease nightmare. Many sugars and sugar products are made from GMO sugar beets. GMO foods have been shown to cause cancer in rats.

Sugar contributes to diabetes, high blood pressure, arthritis, obesity, and cancer. Sugar is a cationic, non-electromagnetic acetic food. As stated previously, acetic body metabolism produces intestinal inflammation, "leaky gut" plus free radical cell changes to the blood, body cells, and organs. These changes, and in association with saturated oils, (trans fats and mega trans) plus high red meat fats, contribute to many diseases in the body. Add the proliferation of candida fungus and parasites, and you have a whole team of ISIS militants ready to attack and destroy your health.

Excess sugar can make you obese. It causes extreme fluctuation in your blood sugar. It also creates a condition called "glycation" which causes damage to your body's blood, body cells, organs, skin, arteries, and joints. It raises the triglycerides in your blood and weakens your immune system by slowing the production of white blood cells. The final blow is that sugar increases the candida, bad bacteria, parasites, and chances to get cancer.

ELECTROMAGNETIC
GOOD DIET VOLTAGE
(pH) 5.6-6.0

NUTRITIONAL VALUE
[1]

[-5]
(50- -5 Cationic)

French Fries, Doughnuts, and Deep-Fried Foods

Most restaurants use grocery omega 6 vegetable "dead" oils from the grocery shelf for cooking. This means for deep frying French fries and all other fried foods. These grocery shelf oils, all non-electromagnetic "dead' oils, change to trans fats and mega trans when used over and over for cooking or deep frying. Trans fats and mega trans when consumed, will cause intestinal inflammation, leaky gut, and free radical damage to blood, body cells, and organs. These damages can raise triglycerides, cholesterol, and cause autoimmune diseases, HBP, heart disease, strokes, arthritis, inflammatory bowel disease, leukocytosis, cancer, and many other diseases. They also increase candida fungus in a person's gut, which many now have shown to be associated with cancer.

Why are these fats so harmful? It is because they have no electrical charge and conduction. In the body they are "dead," non-electromagnetic acetic compounds that lower the blood, body cells, saliva, and urine pH plus causes acidity in the blood, body cells, and organs. Acidity mixed with trans fats and mega trans in the blood can cause the formation of "homocysteine," a clotting substance (sometimes called sticky blood) that is responsible for HBP, blood clots, strokes, and heart attacks. This is why I suggest that a person eat deep-fried foods sparingly or not at all.

As I stated before, Catherine Shanahan, M.D, a heart specialist in Canada, researched and studied 225 stroke and heart attack victims who were just admitted to her hospital, 24 hours or less before. She discovered that 90 percent of these patients had consumed fried or deep-fried "dead" vegetable oils within 24 hours before being admitted to the hospital. These "dead" oils are so vicious because they "spike" the omega 6 to omega 3 ratio from normal, 2:1 or 3:1, to 30:1, and even can spike up to 50:1. The consumption of chronic high sugar, saturated trans fat, and mega trans oil diet is very mean to your blood, body cells, and organs. This is why I recommend people shy away from vegetable oils on the grocery shelf, French fries, and deep-fried foods.

| ELECTROMAGNETIC GOOD DIET VOLTAGE (pH) 5.6-6.0 | NUTRITIONAL VALUE [1] | [-5] (50 - -5 Cationic) |

Sausage, Wieners, and Processed Meats

Deep-fried processed meats, bacon, ham, sausages, wieners, and other processed meats contain the same types of "trans fats" and "mega trans" mentioned before, plus added nitrates and preservatives. They are not good for a person's health.

Although ham, sausage, and wieners are fast to prepare and great for picnics, the omega - 6 "trans fats" and nitrates override all the good taste and protein in the food.

I wish I could say some good things about these good-tasting foods, but there are many negative nutrient problems present. These processed foods contain a substance called mycotoxins, also nitrates, chemical preservatives, omega - 6 oils, and many times honey, sugar, or corn syrup coatings. Chronic use will also increase your type 2 diabetes risk, plus high blood pressure, intestinal inflammation, autoimmune diseases, and free radical cell damage.

Most processed meats change your omega 6 to omega 3 ratio to a much higher omega 6, omega 3 ratio. Very high ratios can initiate strokes and heart attacks, especially in people with high blood pressure and/or excessive homocysteine in their blood. As good as these meats taste, I recommend that you enjoy these foods, but rarely and in moderation. It is hard to refuse a good ham, hot dog, or sausage, especially on holidays or at picnics.

However, I advise you to eat sparingly, and please remember that these foods have no food value, lower your acidity, contain harmful trans fats, and are non-electromagnetic food.

ELECTROMAGNETIC
GOOD DIET VOLTAGE
(pH) 5.6-6.0

NUTRITIONAL VALUE
[1]

[-5]

(50- -5 Cationic)

Diet Drinks, Aspartame, Preservatives, Stevia, and Sugar Substitutes

If Hercules can lift a one-ton rock, it would be no less of a feat than what the pancreas has to perform in the body. The tiny pancreas (less than the size of a baseball) produces six or more hormones and digestive enzymes to help digest our food and drinks. Some of these wonderful digestive enzymes are protease, which digests protein, amylase, which digests carbohydrates, lipase, which digests oils and fats, the insulin that digests sugar and sugar products, plus bromalin, peptides, and polypeptides, used in digestion and absorption of nutrients.

The pancreas can produce only enough insulin to digest about three to four ounces of sugar at one time, even though the average daily consumption of sugar is about 22 ounces per day. You can understand the congestion. With meat or protein, the pancreas can produce enough protease to digest about four ounces of protein, even though some people order a 12-ounce steak at one time. Amylase enzyme also is limited in breaking down excess carbohydrates. Unless you are running in a 26.2-mile marathon, you can see why there is much-undigested food leftover, creating a sugar, blood, gall bladder, liver traffic jam, and/or a protein, blood, and pancreas jam. Diet drinks, sugar substitutes, and preservatives also increase the traffic jam for the pancreas. Many times it cannot produce enough digestive enzymes to digest these products. The excess is not going to end up finding a good destination, as the toxins overload the liver, pancreas, and gall bladder. The excess undigested products cause a serious problem that creates diabetes and high blood pressure in the body.

Sugar substitutes and diet colas also create a real problem as they end up being dangerous toxins that the liver has to contend with. When these toxins in the blood overload the intestinal bacteria and the liver, they just go around in the blood and are dropped off to do damage to the body cells and organs. Diet colas are more damaging than colas with sugar.

ELECTROMAGNETIC
GOOD DIET VOLTAGE
(pH) 5.6-6.2

NUTRITIONAL VALUE
[1]

[-5]

(50 - -5 Cationic)

Cancer and Candida Fungus

Cancer is the leading cause of death in many countries. The U.S. is probably at the top of that list. About 1,800 people in the U.S. die from cancer every day and the death rates are rapidly rising. It is estimated that one out of every two men will have cancer, and one out of every three women will have cancer in their lifetime.

Due to the corrupt drug companies, FDA, and cancer physicians, the cure rate for cancer has not been lowered much in over 60 years, since Otto Warburg found the cause of cancer. Recently, 77 alternative cancer treatment doctors have mysteriously died in the U.S. Many of them even cured cancer with better success rates than the cancer doctors did with conventional treatment. For cancer oncologists, using the conventional methods of chemo, radiation, and surgery, their treatment is a 180 to 200 billion dollar per year bonanza. Unfortunately, their treatment in many tumors usually only treats the symptoms rather than the cause. Chemotherapy and drugs only have about a 55 to 60% chance of curing cancer.

The average oncologist's recovery and cure rate (all cancers) for patients living more than five years, is overall, a little more than 55 percent.

Chemo and radiation destroy both the good body cells with the cancer cells. Since there are two types of cancer cells, regular cancer cells, and stem cells, the radiation and surgery usually kill the regular cancer cells but in many tumors, the stem cells do not die. Often, after submission, the cancer stem cells lay dormant for about two years. they then spring back to life, metastasizing and spreading the tumor.

Cancer usually occurs when a person has a weak immune system where good intestinal bacteria have been infested with bad bacteria, candida fungus, and sometimes, parasites. It usually begins with the diet, when a person has a chronic acetic, non-electromagnetic, low pH system that has lingered over a long period. Sugar, omega 6 oils, and saturated "trans fats" and "mega trans' are very guilty suspects of being straight in the middle of the arena. Some of the other criminals are excessive red meat and carbohydrates, plus an overload of protein, vegetable oil, and sugar which overwhelms the pancreas. The pancreas does not have enough pancreatic enzymes to digest all of the excess foods. . Dr, JoAnna Budwig, Dr. William Kelley, the Gerson clinic, and Dr. Nicholas Gonzalez have cured more than 40,000 cancer patients with alternative cancer treatment. They state that a diet high in raw fresh foods, high electromagnetic foods, hyperthermia, detoxification, an enzyme protocol plus coffee enemas are some of the main cancer treatments. Dr. Budwig also reinforced the pancreatic enzyme deficiency, plus found that candida, sometimes parasites, sticky (homocysteine) blood, and oxygen deprivation are present in almost all cancers.

Recent research has also shown that over 80% of all cancers are associated with candida fungus. It is a bad hombre.

If you want to prevent cancer, change your diet! Other good treatment habits are:

1. Eat very little red meat, eat mostly fowl and fish, or vegetarian.

2. Eliminate all or almost all sugars, sugar substitutes, and pastries. Reduce other carbs, as they have gluten and turn to sugar in the intestinal tract.

3. Eat mostly high electromagnetic ionic raw (live) foods, with plenty of fiber. These must include Jo Anna Budwig's

formula five to seven times a week, plus seven to eleven raw fresh vegetables and fruits daily.

4. Reduce and cut down on all non-electromagnet, acetic, low pH refined, and processed (dead) foods.

5. Substitute red meat with raw almonds, pecans, walnuts, and pistachios.

6. Consume only flaxseed and omega-3 oils and stay away from deep-fried foods.

7. Do not use any oil found on the grocery shelf.

8. Use coconut oil, palm oil, or butter for cooking.

9. Be sure to take, vitamin C, 1,000 to 2,000 mg/day, D3, 15,000 to 20,000 IUs/day, magnesium, zinc, turmeric and L-arginine.

10. Get and take three to five wobenzym-N (pancreatic) tablets every day.

11. Don't get stressed out. Stress is one of the important causes of cancer.

12. With low pH, take 6 – 10 barley tablets a day. Also take a cucumber, watermelon, and water to raise pH to alkaline. Check urine, saliva/w pH paper every morning and night.

13. Have a meditation time or find a relaxation time for you. Know that God is with you.

Take time out to enjoy this wonderful, great, exciting world and the outdoors, relative gatherings, the theatre, books, television, and the computer. 15. We live in the greatest era of all time. Remember to dream, work hard, learn, and enjoy this wonderful world and universe

ELECTROMAGNETIC GOOD DIET VOLTAGE (pH) 5.6-6.2

NUTRITIONAL VALUE [-15]

[-15]

(100 - 50 Ionic)

(50 to -15 Cationic)

The Importance of Great Intestinal Bacteria

One of the most vital and important systems in your body is your small intestine and intestinal bacteria. For every cell in your body, you have ten or more intestinal bacteria or 25+ trillion of the little creatures. These 25+ trillion bacteria are responsible for your digestion, cell and organ function, energy and immune system, health plus, believe it or not, a part of your mental functions.

The health of your intestinal bacteria is your responsibility. Many people eat a poor diet. They treat their bacteria like the prisoners of Roman soldiers. What you eat determines the ratio of good to bad bacteria in your gut. That ratio of the two and one half to four pounds of bacteria should be 80 percent or higher of good ones, and 20 percent or less of bad ones. With a great diet, your healthy ratio should stay around 80 percent good and 20 percent bad bacteria. That is not always the case with a bad diet.

When you eat a majority of acetic or low pH, non-electromagnetic (dead) food and oils, or accidentally get some parasites, toxic chemicals, or metals, the good to bad bacteria ratio can change. The good to bad ratio may get out of synch, or change to 70 percent to 30 percent or maybe worse, depending on your diet and how many refined, acetic, non-electromagnetic foods you consume.

With a poor, non-electromagnetic, low acetic pH diet with bad bacteria, candida fungus, and parasites, great toxins are created in the small intestines. They irritate the gut lining. They create inflammation toxins. Worse yet, the toxins are harmful, health-destroying, including acetaldehyde and other acetic toxins. These toxins and other criminals erode the lining of the small intestine, causing gut inflammation and holes, called "leaky" gut. The resulting leaky gut refers to the holes produced by the toxins which allow bad food toxins, bad bacteria, food particles, protein, and other gangsters into the blood. This results in autoimmune and other body, organ, and brain diseases.

ELECTROMAGNETIC
GOOD DIET VOLTAGE
(pH) 6.2-6.4

NUTRITIONAL VALUE

[15]

[100]

(100 – 50 Ionic)

www.ingramcontent.com/pod-product-compliance
Lightning Source LLC
Chambersburg PA
CBHW062125020426
42335CB00013B/1098